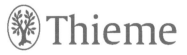

# Instrumentation for Minimally Invasive Spine Surgery

**Kern Singh, MD**
Professor
Department of Orthopaedic Surgery
Co-Director
Minimally Invasive Spine Institute
Rush University Medical Center
Chicago, Illinois

332 illustrations

Thieme
New York • Stuttgart • Delhi • Rio de Janeiro

Library of Congress Cataloging-in-Publication Data is available with the publisher

**Important note:** Medicine is an ever-changing science undergoing continual development. Research and clinical experience are continually expanding our knowledge, in particular our knowledge of proper treatment and drug therapy. Insofar as this book mentions any dosage or application, readers may rest assured that the authors, editors, and publishers have made every effort to ensure that such references are in accordance with **the state of knowledge at the time of production of the book.**

Nevertheless, this does not involve, imply, or express any guarantee or responsibility on the part of the publishers in respect to any dosage instructions and forms of applications stated in the book. **Every user is requested to examine carefully** the manufacturers' leaflets accompanying each drug and to check, if necessary in consultation with a physician or specialist, whether the dosage schedules mentioned therein or the contraindications stated by the manufacturers differ from the statements made in the present book. Such examination is particularly important with drugs that are either rarely used or have been newly released on the market. Every dosage schedule or every form of application used is entirely at the user's own risk and responsibility. The authors and publishers request every user to report to the publishers any discrepancies or inaccuracies noticed. If errors in this work are found after publication, errata will be posted at www.thieme.com on the product description page.

Some of the product names, patents, and registered designs referred to in this book are in fact registered trademarks or proprietary names even though specific reference to this fact is not always made in the text. Therefore, the appearance of a name without designation as proprietary is not to be construed as a representation by the publisher that it is in the public domain.

© 2021. Thieme. All rights reserved.

Thieme Medical Publishers, Inc.
333 Seventh Avenue, New York, NY 10001 USA
+1 800 782 3488, customerservice@thieme.com

Cover design: Thieme Publishing Group
Typesetting by DiTech Process Solutions, India

Printed in USA by King Printing Company, Inc.   5 4 3 2 1

ISBN 978-1-62623-202-0

Also available as an e-book:
eISBN 978-1-62623-203-7

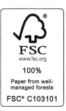

*I dedicate this book to my parents. We did not have much, but it sure felt like a lot.*
*I look back and treasure those memories. It is amazing how much has changed, but those values I grew up with remain the same.*

# Contents

Preface . . . . . . . . . . . . . . . . . . . . . . . . . . . . . . . . . . . . . . . . . . . . . . . . . . . . . . . . . . . xi

Acknowledgments . . . . . . . . . . . . . . . . . . . . . . . . . . . . . . . . . . . . . . . . . . . . . . . xii

Contributors . . . . . . . . . . . . . . . . . . . . . . . . . . . . . . . . . . . . . . . . . . . . . . . . . . . . xiii

List of Abbreviations . . . . . . . . . . . . . . . . . . . . . . . . . . . . . . . . . . . . . . . . . . . . . xiv

1. Minimally Invasive Spinal Instrumentation: Past, Present, and Future . . . 1
   Benjamin Khechen, Britany E. Haws, Kaitlyn L. Cardinal, Jordan A. Guntin, and Kern Singh

Part I  Posterior Approach

2. Introduction to MIS Posterior Approach . . . . . . . . . . . . . . . . . . . . . . . . . . . . . . . 4
   Benjamin Khechen, Brittany E. Haws, Ankur Narain, Fady Hijji, Jordan A. Guntin,
   Kaitlyn L. Cardinal, and Kern Singh

| | | | | | |
|---|---|---|---|---|---|
| 2.1 | Introduction . . . . . . . . . . . . . . . . . . . | 4 | 2.3.3 | Disk Space Preparation . . . . . . . . . . . . | 5 |
| | | | 2.3.4 | Interbody Cage Placement . . . . . . . . . | 6 |
| 2.2 | Surgical Anatomy . . . . . . . . . . . . . . . . | 4 | 2.3.5 | Supplemental Fixation . . . . . . . . . . . . | 6 |
| 2.3 | Surgical Technique . . . . . . . . . . . . . | 4 | 2.3.6 | Closure and Postoperative Care . . . . . . | 8 |
| | | | 2.3.7 | Complications . . . . . . . . . . . . . . . . . . . . | 8 |
| 2.3.1 | Positioning . . . . . . . . . . . . . . . . . . . . . . | 4 | 2.3.8 | Outcomes . . . . . . . . . . . . . . . . . . . . . . . | 9 |
| 2.3.2 | Approach (Exposure) for MIS Transforaminal Lumbar Interbody Fusion . . . . . . . . . . . . . . . . . . . . . . . . . | 4 | | | |

3. Posterior Retractor Systems . . . . . . . . . . . . . . . . . . . . . . . . . . . . . . . . . . . . . . . 11
   Mohammed Abbas, Benjamin Khechen, Brittany E. Haws, Ankur S. Narain, Fady Hijji,
   Kaitlyn L. Cardinal, Jordan A. Guntin, and Kern Singh

| | | | | | |
|---|---|---|---|---|---|
| 3.1 | Introduction . . . . . . . . . . . . . . . . . . . | 11 | 3.3 | Expandable Retractor Systems . . . | 17 |
| 3.1.1 | Retractor Components . . . . . . . . . . . . | 11 | 3.3.1 | Flat Blade . . . . . . . . . . . . . . . . . . . . . . . | 21 |
| 3.1.2 | Types of Retraction Systems . . . . . . . . | 11 | 3.4 | Pedicle-Screw–Based Retractor |
| 3.1.3 | Complications . . . . . . . . . . . . . . . . . . . . | 12 | | Systems . . . . . . . . . . . . . . . . . . . . . . . | 22 |
| 3.2 | Static Retractor Systems . . . . . . . . | 13 | | | |

4. Posterior Interbody Cages . . . . . . . . . . . . . . . . . . . . . . . . . . . . . . . . . . . . . . . . . 26
   Adam B. Wiggins, Benjamin Khechen, Brittany E. Haws, Ankur S. Narain, Fady Hijji,
   Kamran Movassaghi, Kaitlyn L. Cardinal, Jordan A. Guntin, and Kern Singh

| | | | | | |
|---|---|---|---|---|---|
| 4.1 | Introduction . . . . . . . . . . . . . . . . . . . | 26 | 4.2 | Static Carbon Fiber Interbody |
| 4.1.1 | Interbody Cage Overview . . . . . . . . . . | 26 | | Cages . . . . . . . . . . . . . . . . . . . . . . . . . | 29 |
| 4.1.2 | Interbody Cage Classification . . . . . . . | 26 | 4.3 | Static Metal Interbody Cages . . . . | 48 |
| 4.1.3 | Minimally Invasive Transforaminal Lumbar Interbody Fusion . . . . . . . . . . | 28 | | | |

# Contents

**4.4** Static Mixed Composition Interbody Cages ............... 57

**4.5** Static Allograft Interbody Cages .. 63

**4.6** Expandable Interbody Cages .... 66

**5. Percutaneous Pedicle Screw Systems** ................................... 73

*Simon P. Lalehzarian, Benjamin Khechen, Brittany E. Haws, Jordan A. Guntin, Kaitlyn L. Cardinal, and Kern Singh*

**5.1** Introduction ................... 73

5.1.1 Pedicle Screw Components ........ 73
5.1.2 Pedicle Screw Constructs .......... 75

5.1.3 Complications .................... 75

**5.2 Percutaneous Pedicle Screw Systems** ........................ 76

**6. Cortical Screw Systems** ..................................................... 88

*Simon P. Lalehzarian, Benjamin Khechen, Brittany E. Haws, Kaitlyn L. Cardinal, Jordan A. Guntin, Sravisht Iyer, and Kern Singh*

**6.1** Introduction ................... 88

6.1.1 Components .................... 88

6.1.2 Efficacy and Complications ........ 89

**6.2 Cortical Screw Systems** ......... 90

**7. Facet Screw Systems** ....................................................... 96

*Simon P. Lalehzarian, Benjamin Khechen, Brittany E. Haws, Kaitlyn L. Cardinal, Jordan A. Guntin, and Kern Singh*

**7.1** Introduction ................... 96

7.1.1 Facet Screw Components .......... 96

7.1.2 Outcomes ....................... 96

**7.2 Facet Screw Systems** ........... 98

**8. Spinous Process Fixation Systems** ........................................ 104

*Jordan A. Guntin, Benjamin Khechen, Brittany E. Haws, Kaitlyn L. Cardinal, and Kern Singh*

**8.1** Introduction ................... 104

8.1.1 Interspinous Fixation Device Components ................... 104

8.1.2 Outcomes ....................... 105

**8.2 Spinous Process Fixation Systems** ...................... 106

## Part II  Lateral Approach

**9. Introduction to MIS Lateral Approach** ................................... 120

*Sravisht Iyer, Benjamin Khechen, Brittany E. Haws, Jordan A. Guntin, Kaitlyn L. Cardinal, and Kern Singh*

**9.1** Introduction ................... 120

**9.2** Surgical Anatomy .............. 120

**9.3** Surgical Technique ........... 120

9.3.1 Positioning .................... 120
9.3.2 Approach ....................... 121

9.3.3 Disk Space Preparation .......... 122
9.3.4 Interbody Cage Placement ........ 122
9.3.5 Supplemental Fixation .......... 123
9.3.6 Closure ........................ 123

**9.4 Complications** ................. 123

**9.5 Outcomes** ..................... 124

**10.** **Lateral Retractor Systems** ................................................. 126

*Mohammed Abbas, Benjamin Khechen, Brittany E. Haws, Jordan A. Guntin,*
*Kaitlyn L. Cardinal, and Kern Singh*

**10.1** **Introduction** .................. 126    **10.2** **Lateral Retractor Systems** ...... 126

**11.** **Lateral Interbody Cages** ................................................... 133

*Adam B. Wiggins, Benjamin Khechen, Brittany E. Haws, Jordan A. Guntin, Kaitlyn L. Cardinal,*
*Eric H. Lamoutte, and Kern Singh*

**11.1** **Introduction** .................. 133    **11.4** **Static Mixed Composition**
         **Interbody Cages** .............. 139
**11.2** **Static PEEK Lateral Interbody**
      **Cages** ......................... 133    **11.5** **Expandable Interbody Cages** ... 142

**11.3** **Static Metal Interbody Cages** ... 138

**12.** **Lateral Fixation Systems** .................................................. 145

*Simon P. Lalehzarian, Benjamin Khechen, Brittany E. Haws, Kaitlyn L. Cardinal, Jordan A. Guntin,*
*Eric H. Lamoutte, and Kern Singh*

**12.1** **Introduction** .................. 145    **12.3** **Lateral Fixation Device**
         **Systems** ...................... 146
**12.2** **Outcomes** ..................... 145

**13.** **Vertebral Body Replacement Devices** ..................................... 156

*Simon P. Lalehzarian, Benjamin Khechen, Brittany E. Haws, Kaitlyn L. Cardinal, Jordan A. Guntin,*
*Eric H. Lamoutte, and Kern Singh*

**13.1** **Introduction** .................. 156    **13.4** **Expandable Carbon Fiber VBR**
         **Devices** ....................... 166
13.1.1 Vertebral Body Replacement Device
       Classification .................... 156    **13.5** **Expandable Metal VBR**
13.1.2 Efficacy and Outcomes .......... 158          **Devices** ....................... 171
**13.2** **Static PEEK VBR Devices** ....... 160

**13.3** **Static Metal VBR Devices** ....... 164

**Part III** **Other**

**14.** **Percutaneous Cement Augmentation Systems** ......................... 180

*Kaitlyn L. Cardinal, Benjamin Khechen, Brittany E. Haws, Jordan A. Guntin, Sravisht Iyer, and*
*Kern Singh*

**14.1** **Introduction** .................. 180    14.1.3 Complications ................... 182
         **14.2** **Percutaneous Cement**
14.1.1 Components .................... 180          **Augmentation Systems** ........ 183
14.1.2 Outcomes ...................... 181

# Contents

**15.** **Biologics** ............................................................ 191

*Kaitlyn L. Cardinal, Benjamin Khechen, Brittany E. Haws, Jordan A. Guntin, Sravisht Iyer, and Kern Singh*

**15.1** **Introduction**................... 191

15.1.1 Biologics Classification ........... 191
15.1.2 Outcomes....................... 192
15.1.3 Complications................... 193

**15.2** **Bone Ceramics**................ 193

**15.3** **Demineralized Bone Matrix** .... 204

**15.4** **Structural Allograft**........... 213

**16.** **Surgical Navigation Systems** ............................................... 218

*Simon P. Lalehzarian, Benjamin Khechen, Brittany E. Haws, Kaitlyn L. Cardinal, Jordan A. Guntin, and Kern Singh*

**16.1** **Introduction**................... 218

**16.2** **Components**................... 218

16.2.1 Imaging Modalities .............. 218
16.2.2 Workstation ................... 218

16.2.3 Dynamic Reference Frames........ 219
16.2.4 Surgical Navigation Instruments ... 219
**16.3** **Outcomes** .................... 219

**16.4** **Surgical Navigation Systems** ... 221

**Index** ............................................................. 224

# Preface

As the field of minimally invasive spine surgery rapidly evolves, so do the medical devices and technology that facilitate these procedures. Different devices can be tailored to a particular surgical need with respect to procedure type or approach. Their integration with the use of minimally invasive techniques has allowed surgeons to tackle more complex spinal pathologies and generate new ways to improve clinical outcomes. While these advances can extend the capabilities of surgeons and provide elevated patient care, the huge variety of devices available can be daunting.

To help surgeons navigate these many options, this text combines a thorough review of empirical literature with expert experience and manufacturer specifications to detail the advantages and capabilities of a wide variety of unique devices. The technology discussed include retractor systems, interbody cages, and fixation systems for both posterior and lateral approaches, as well as cements, biologics, and surgical navigation systems. We hope that this book will serve as a valuable resource for minimally invasive spine surgeons as they consider the improvements that available devices may bring to their practice and patients.

*Kern Singh, MD*

# Acknowledgments

I dedicate this book to my countless research team members. I hope that one day when you are in a position to help someone else out you do the same. Nothing is more rewarding than seeing all of you work so hard and accomplish so much. Truly inspiring.

*Kern Singh, MD*

# Contributors

**Mohammed Abbas, MD**
Resident Physician
Department of Orthopaedic Surgery
Rush University Medical Center
Chicago, Illinois

**Kaitlyn L. Cardinal, BS**
Medical Student
Department of Orthopaedic Surgery
Rush University Medical Center
Chicago, Illinois

**Jordan A. Guntin, BS**
Medical Student
Department of Orthopaedic Surgery
Rush University Medical Center
Chicago, Illinois

**Britany E. Haws, MD**
Resident Physician
Department of Orthopaedics and Rehabilitation
University of Rochester
Rochester, New York

**Fady Hijji, MD**
Resident Physician
Department of Orthopaedic Surgery
Wright State University Boonshoft School of
    Medicine
Dayton, Ohio

**Sravisht Iyer, MD**
Assistant Attending Physician
Department of Orthopaedic Surgery
Hospital for Special Surgery
New York, New York

**Benjamin Khechen, MD**
Resident Physician
Department of Orthopaedic Surgery
Rush University Medical Center
Chicago, Illinois

**Simon P. Lalehzarian, MS**
Medical Student
Department of Orthopaedic Surgery
Rush University Medical Center
Chicago, Illinois

**Eric H. Lamoutte, BS**
Medical Student
Department of Orthopaedic Surgery
Rush University Medical Center
Chicago, Illinois

**Kamran Movassaghi, MD**
Resident Physician
Department of Orthopaedic Surgery
UCSF Fresno
Fresno, California

**Ankur S. Narain, MD**
Resident Physician
Department of Orthopaedic Surgery
UMass Memorial Medical Center
Worcester, Massachusetts

**Kern Singh, MD**
Professor
Department of Orthopaedic Surgery
Co-Director
Minimally Invasive Spine Institute
Rush University Medical Center
Chicago, Illinois

**Adam B. Wiggins, MD**
Resident Physician
Department of Orthopaedic Surgery
Rush University Medical Center
Chicago, Illinois

# List of Abbreviations

| | | | |
|---|---|---|---|
| 2D | two-dimensional | ODI | Oswestry Disability Index |
| 3D | three-dimensional | PEEK | polyetheretherketone |
| ALIF | anterior lumbar interbody fusion | PLF | posterolateral fusion |
| AN | anatomically narrow | PLIF | posterior lumbar interbody fusion |
| AP | anteroposterior | PMMA | polymethyl methacrylate |
| BMP | bone morphogenic protein | RPM | reverse phase medium |
| CFRP | carbon fiber reinforced polymer | rhBMP-2 | recombinant human bone morpho-genic protein-2 |
| CT | computed tomography | | |
| DBM | demineralized bone matrix | SF-36 | 36-Item Short Form Survey |
| EMG | electromyogram/electromyographic | TCP | tricalcium phosphate |
| HA | hydroxyapatite | TGF-β | transforming growth factor-beta |
| HC | horizontal cylinder | TLIF | transforaminal lumbar interbody fusion |
| iCT | intraoperative CT | | |
| IFD | interspinous fixation device | TPS | Titanium Plasma Spray |
| iGA | Integrated Global Alignment | VAS | Visual Analog Scale |
| LLIF | lateral lumbar interbody fusion | VBB | Vertebral Body Balloon |
| LO | Large Oblique | VBR | vertebral body replacement |
| MIDLF | midline lumbar fusion | VCF | vertebral compression fractures |
| MIS | minimally invasive surgery | VR | vertical ring |
| MPF | Modular Plate Fixation | XLIF | eXtreme lateral interbody fusion |
| OB | open box | | |

# 1 Minimally Invasive Spinal Instrumentation: Past, Present, and Future

*Benjamin Khechen, Britany E. Haws, Kaitlyn L. Cardinal, Jordan A. Guntin, and Kern Singh*

In recent decades, technological advances in minimally invasive spine (MIS) surgery have revolutionized the surgical management of spinal pathology. The primary goal of MIS remains the improvement of postoperative outcomes and patient satisfaction. Compared to "traditional" open approaches, MIS techniques have demonstrated reduced intraoperative blood loss, shortened length of inpatient stay, decreased complications, and reduced postoperative pain and narcotics consumption.[1,2,3,4] MIS approaches in spine surgery have proven to be cost-effective through the reduction of morbidity and enhanced utility in ambulatory surgical centers.[5,6,7,8] Furthermore, MIS surgery has provided a surgical option for elderly patients deemed inappropriate surgical candidates for open procedures.[9,10,11,12]

The modern MIS surgery era was launched in 1997, with the first reported microendoscopic diskectomy published by Foley and Smith.[13] This was followed in 2001 by Foley's novel technique to pass rods percutaneously using an arc-based approach.[14] In the ensuing years, the first reports of MIS fusion techniques were published, including MIS posterior lumbar interbody fusion in 2002[15] and MIS transforaminal lumbar interbody fusion in 2006.[16] MIS approaches have since been developed for several conditions including degenerative, deformity, and oncologic pathology.[9,10,11,12,17,18]

A promising future truly exists for MIS surgery. New technologies are now being developed with the specific intention of use in MIS surgery. Greater attention has been placed on surgical navigation systems that provide improved accuracy in screw placement.[19,20,21] The role of intraoperative image guidance will continue to evolve in MIS surgery, particularly as technological advances make these systems more adaptable and cost-effective. However, spine surgeons must retain a level of sensibility when considering the use of these new technologies in MIS surgery. As with all surgical techniques, a learning curve exists for MIS surgery. As such, these techniques must be comprehensively taught in residency programs to better equip future spine surgeons.

This text is intended to provide a comprehensive overview of current MIS instrumentation for senior spine surgeons, spine surgeons in training, and surgical assistants. Section 1 details instrumentation utilized in MIS posterior approach, followed by Section 2, which details instrumentation used in lateral MIS approach. Section 3 provides information on current biologics and surgical navigation systems used in MIS surgery. We would like to extend our appreciation to the spinal device companies that have agreed to participate in our textbook.

## References

[1] Wang MY, Lerner J, Lesko J, McGirt MJ. Acute hospital costs after minimally invasive versus open lumbar interbody fusion: data from a US national database with 6106 patients. J Spinal Disord Tech. 2012; 25(6):324–328

[2] Mobbs RJ, Li J, Sivabalan P, Raley D, Rao PJ. Outcomes after decompressive laminectomy for lumbar spinal stenosis: comparison between minimally invasive unilateral laminectomy for bilateral decompression and open laminectomy: clinical article. J Neurosurg Spine. 2014; 21(2):179–186

[3] Skovrlj B, Belton P, Zarzour H, Qureshi SA. Perioperative outcomes in minimally invasive lumbar spine surgery: a systematic review. World J Orthop. 2015; 6(11):996–1005

[4] Singh K, Nandyala SV, Marquez-Lara A, et al. A perioperative cost analysis comparing single-level minimally invasive and open transforaminal lumbar interbody fusion. Spine J. 2014; 14(8):1694–1701

[5] Oppenheimer JH, DeCastro I, McDonnell DE. Minimally invasive spine technology and minimally invasive spine surgery: a historical review. Neurosurg Focus. 2009; 27(3):E9

[6] Best NM, Sasso RC. Success and safety in outpatient microlumbar discectomy. J Spinal Disord Tech. 2006; 19(5):334–337

[7] Helseth Ø, Lied B, Halvorsen CM, Ekseth K, Helseth E. Outpatient cervical and lumbar spine surgery is feasible and safe: a consecutive single center series of 1449 patients. Neurosurgery. 2015; 76(6):728–737, discussion 737–738

[8] Walid MS, Robinson JS, III, Robinson ER, Brannick BB, Ajjan M, Robinson JS, Jr. Comparison of outpatient and inpatient spine surgery patients with regards to obesity, comorbidities and readmission for infection. J Clin Neurosci. 2010; 17(12):1497–1498

[9] Khan NR, Clark AJ, Lee SL, Venable GT, Rossi NB, Foley KT. Surgical outcomes for minimally invasive vs open transforaminal lumbar interbody fusion: an updated systematic review and meta-analysis. Neurosurgery. 2015; 77(6):847–874, discussion 874

[10] Phan K, Rao PJ, Kam AC, Mobbs RJ. Minimally invasive versus open transforaminal lumbar interbody fusion for treatment of degenerative lumbar disease: systematic review and meta-analysis. Eur Spine J. 2015; 24(5):1017–1030

[11] Soliman HM. Irrigation endoscopic decompressive laminotomy. A new endoscopic approach for spinal stenosis decompression. Spine J. 2015; 15(10):2282–2289

[12] Patel VV, Whang PG, Haley TR, et al. Superion interspinous process spacer for intermittent neurogenic claudication secondary to moderate lumbar spinal stenosis: two-year results from a randomized controlled FDA-IDE pivotal trial. Spine. 2015; 40(5):275–282

[13] Foley KT, Smith MM. Microendoscopic discectomy. Tech Neurosurg. 1997; 3:301–307

[14] Foley KT, Gupta SK, Justis JR, Sherman MC. Percutaneous pedicle screw fixation of the lumbar spine. Neurosurg Focus. 2001; 10(4):E10

[15] Khoo LT, Palmer S, Laich DT, Fessler RG. Minimally invasive percutaneous posterior lumbar interbody fusion. Neurosurgery. 2002; 51(5) Suppl:S166–S181

[16] Holly LT, Schwender JD, Rouben DP, Foley KT. Minimally invasive transforaminal lumbar interbody fusion: indications, technique, and complications. Neurosurg Focus. 2006; 20(3):E6

[17] Anand N, Baron EM, Thaiyananthan G, Khalsa K, Goldstein TB. Minimally invasive multilevel percutaneous correction and fusion for adult lumbar degenerative scoliosis: a technique and feasibility study. J Spinal Disord Tech. 2008; 21(7):459–467

[18] Lall RR, Smith ZA, Wong AP, Miller D, Fessler RG. Minimally invasive thoracic corpectomy: surgical strategies for malignancy, trauma, and complex spinal pathologies. Minim Invasive Surg. 2012; 2012:213791

[19] Cho JY, Chan CK, Lee SH, Lee HY. The accuracy of 3D image navigation with a cutaneously fixed dynamic reference frame in minimally invasive transforaminal lumbar interbody fusion. Comput Aided Surg. 2012; 17(6):300–309

[20] Ebmeier K, Giest K, Kalff R. Intraoperative computerized tomography for improved accuracy of spinal navigation in pedicle screw placement of the thoracic spine. Acta Neurochir Suppl (Wien). 2003; 85:105–113

[21] Kim CW, Lee YP, Taylor W, Oygar A, Kim WK. Use of navigation-assisted fluoroscopy to decrease radiation exposure during minimally invasive spine surgery. Spine J. 2008; 8(4):584–590

# Part I

## Posterior Approach

2    Introduction to MIS
Posterior Approach     *4*

3    Posterior Retractor
Systems     *11*

4    Posterior Interbody
Cages     *26*

5    Percutaneous Pedicle
Screw Systems     *73*

6    Cortical Screw Systems     *88*

7    Facet Screw Systems     *96*

8    Spinous Process Fixation Systems     *104*

# 2 Introduction to MIS Posterior Approach

Benjamin Khechen, Brittany E. Haws, Ankur Narain, Fady Hijji, Jordan A. Guntin, Kaitlyn L. Cardinal, and Kern Singh

## 2.1 Introduction

The minimally invasive spine (MIS) posterior approach for decompression and fusion of the lumbar spine utilizes the Harms modification of the original Wiltse approach, described in 1968.[1,2] The posterior parasagittal technique was designed to reduce the morbidity associated with the traditional open midline approach.[3] This approach minimizes muscular trauma by dissecting the natural plane of two separate muscle groups and allowed for the preservation of midline structures.[3] The MIS posterior approach can be utilized for the treatment of a variety of pathologies of the thoracic and lumbar spine.[4,5] These treatment options can include decompression, diskectomy, posterior instrumentation, and interbody fusion.[4,6] This approach allows for the direct decompression of neural elements and direct access to the disk space.[4,6,7,8]

## 2.2 Surgical Anatomy

The lumbar spinous processes and iliac crests are easily palpable for orientation prior to performing the MIS posterior approach. This approach utilizes the internervous plane between the paraspinal muscles, minimizing any requirement for muscle dissection. However, multiple structures of the posterior vertebrae are encountered with this approach. The lamina and facet joints are directly involved with this approach, and their removal will lead to exposure of the traversing nerve root and underlying dura mater.

Due to the posterior orientation of this approach, some structures are at risk for injury.[4] Primarily, the traversing and exiting nerve roots can be iatrogenically injured as it passes the surgical corridor. Additionally, the dura is within the proximity of the approach and may be inadvertently disrupted while decompressing the overlying structures.

## 2.3 Surgical Technique

### 2.3.1 Positioning

Patients undergoing a posterior MIS approach are placed in the prone position on a radiolucent table following anesthesia induction (▶ Fig. 2.1). Pads are placed under the manubrium and anterior superior iliac spine to maintain lumbar lordosis. The patient's legs are left extended, while the arms are placed in 90 degrees of shoulder and elbow flexion. A foam pad is placed underneath the flexed arms to reduce the risk of ulnar nerve compression. Prior to surgical preparation and draping, fluoroscopic images are obtained of the lumbar spine to confirm visibility of the pedicles and other spinal anatomy.

### 2.3.2 Approach (Exposure) for MIS Transforaminal Lumbar Interbody Fusion

A 22-gauge needle is oriented toward the facet joint at the disk level of interest and inserted. A fluoroscopic image is then obtained to confirm the correct surgical level.

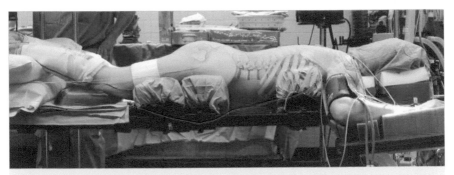

**Fig. 2.1** Demonstration of prone surgical positioning. (Reproduced, with permission, from Singh K, Vaccaro A, eds. Pocket Atlas of Spine Surgery. 2nd ed. New York, NY: Thieme; 2018.)

The side of the operation to be performed is determined by the location of neurologic symptoms. Following confirmation, an incision is made paramedially, 4 to 5 cm lateral to the midline. The incision is made to be approximately 2.0 cm in length in order to fit the final tubular retractor. Bovie cautery is used to incise the underlying fascia. The smallest tubular dilator is inserted through the muscle down to the level of the facet joint or lamina in a lateral to medial direction. Once appropriate positioning of the initial dilator is determined using fluoroscopy, serial dilators are inserted, gradually increasing the size of the surgical corridor. Finally, the tubular retractor is then placed over the last dilator and the dilators are subsequently removed (▶ Fig. 2.2). The tubular retractor is then fixed to the table after being docked over the area of interest. Fluoroscopy is then utilized to confirm adequate positioning and orientation of the retractor.

The following aspects of the procedure are performed under illumination with loupe magnification or with the use of an operating microscope. Residual soft tissue overlying the lamina and facet is removed with electrocautery followed by pituitary instruments. Following laminar exposure, a high-speed drill is used to perform a complete bilateral laminectomy. Bone removed from the laminectomy can be used as graft material within the interbody cage. Once the ligamentum flavum is identified, the laminectomy is extended cranially until the flavum insertion is visualized; however, the flavum is left intact to protect underlying neural structures. Following complete laminectomy, a facetectomy is performed. To facilitate the facetectomy, the inferior articular process and pars interarticularis are removed first. Caution must be taken to avoid drilling into the pedicle. Once the facet joint is removed, the ligamentum is removed to expose the underlying nerve roots. The working zone for MIS transforaminal lumbar interbody fusion (TLIF) is defined medially by the traversing nerve root and laterally by the exiting nerve root (▶ Fig. 2.3). The venous plexus surrounding the epidural space can cause significant bleeding; therefore, adequate hemostasis using bipolar electrocautery is crucial to maintain appropriate visualization of the disk space.

### 2.3.3 Disk Space Preparation

A complete diskectomy is performed through the tubular retractor. Pituitaries and curettes can be utilized to perform the annulotomy and remove disk material. Once all disk material is removed, the intervertebral space is distracted with paddle distractors and the endplates are prepared utilizing end plate shavers.

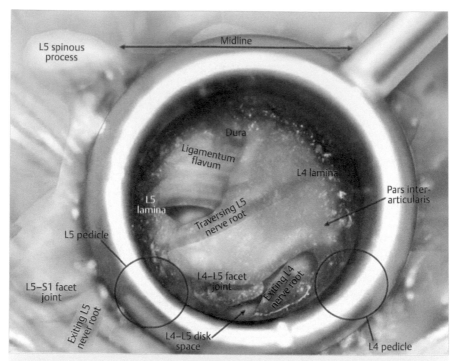

**Fig. 2.2** Initial exposure of the working portal with the corresponding structures. (Reproduced, with permission, from Singh K, Vaccaro A, eds. Pocket Atlas of Spine Surgery. 2nd ed. New York, NY: Thieme; 2018.)

### 2.3.4 Interbody Cage Placement

Trial sizers are placed into the disk space under fluoroscopic guidance to determine the appropriate size for the implant. A bone funnel containing the previously morcellized bone fragments is placed through the disk space. The interbody cage is then impacted into the disk space toward the midline (▶ Fig. 2.4). Care should be taken to protect the nearby nerve root. In select cases, osteobiologic products such as recombinant human bone morphogenetic protein-2 can be utilized with the interbody cage. Bilateral cages can also be inserted using a bilateral approach.

### 2.3.5 Supplemental Fixation

Percutaneous pedicle screws are placed into the adjacent vertebrae of the MIS TLIF to provide supplemental fixation. The steps leading to the insertion of the guidewires are performed prior to retractor placement for the MIS TLIF. The pedicle screws themselves are placed after the completion of the MIS TLIF.

A Jamshidi trocar is inserted onto the center of the pedicle using fluoroscopic guidance. A guidewire is placed through the trocar and advanced until it reaches the medial pedicle wall, as identified by anteroposterior (AP) fluoroscopic images (▶ Fig. 2.5). These steps are repeated for the adjacent level. It is necessary to ensure that the spinous processes are centered in the AP view in order to adequately assess screw placement.

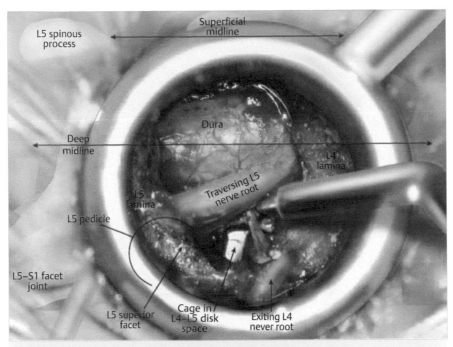

**Fig. 2.3** Exposure following removal of the ligamentum flavum. (Reproduced, with permission, from Singh K, Vaccaro A, eds. Pocket Atlas of Spine Surgery. 2nd ed. New York, NY: Thieme; 2018.)

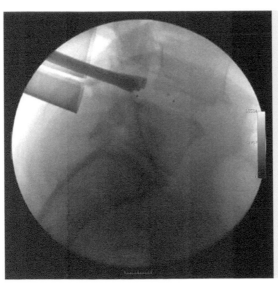

**Fig. 2.4** Lateral fluoroscopic image of the interbody cage being impacted into place. (Reproduced, with permission, from Singh K, Vaccaro A, eds. Pocket Atlas of Spine Surgery. 2nd ed. New York, NY: Thieme; 2018.)

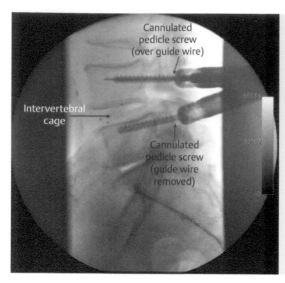

Fig. 2.5 Fluoroscopic image of cannulated pedicle screws upon insertion. (Reproduced, with permission, from Singh K, Vaccaro A, eds. Pocket Atlas of Spine Surgery. 2nd ed. New York, NY: Thieme; 2018.)

Once all guide wires have been placed, a lateral fluoroscopic image is taken to ensure that the guide wires have been advanced past the posterior vertebral body wall. Once correct guide wire placement is confirmed, pedicle screws are inserted using the guide wires. The guide wires are then removed and a rod is inserted, connecting the tulips of the inserted pedicle screws.

## 2.3.6 Closure and Postoperative Care

Final fluoroscopic images are obtained to confirm accurate placement of all implants and instrumentation. The wound is then irrigated and the fascia and skin are subsequently closed in layers. Following the procedure, attempts should be made to mobilize the patient early to maximize functionality postoperatively.

## 2.3.7 Complications

While MIS techniques may exhibit some advantages over traditional techniques, including reduced blood loss, rate of transfusion, postoperative pain, and length of stay, the complications of MIS and open posterior approaches remain similar.[4,9,10,11,12] Primary complications associated with MIS TLIF are dural tear, cerebrospinal fluid leak, neurologic injury/deficits, hemorrhage, pedicle screw malposition, and cage migration.[13] The overall complication rate following MIS TLIF ranges from 0 to 33.3%.[13] Due to the narrow surgical corridor, particular concern has arisen for an increased risk for pseudarthrosis and subsidence following MIS TLIF.[6,14] Wang noted that MIS patients may have an increased risk for cage subsidence due the smaller footprint of MIS interbody implants.[15] However, despite these concerns, many studies and systematic reviews have noted similar or reduced risk for complications following MIS TLIF when compared to open techniques.[15,16,17,18]

The variation in complication rates following MIS TLIF has been attributed to the learning curve associated with MIS techniques.[19,20,21,22] In a review of a single surgeon, Silva et al determined that the 50% learning milestone for MIS TLIF was after the 9th case, and the 90% milestone was after the 39th case.[19] Additionally, the rate of complications reduced substantially from 30 to 20.5% before reaching the 50 and 90% learning milestones, respectively. These findings suggest that surgeon expertise and comfort with the posterior MIS techniques may have an impact on the efficacy of MIS TLIF.

## 2.3.8 Outcomes

Despite the steep learning curve, MIS TLIF has been demonstrated to have favorable outcomes. Previous studies have demonstrated significant improvement in both Visual Analog Scale (VAS) and Oswestry Disability Index (ODI) scores at approximately 2-year follow-up.[23] Additionally, comparative studies between MIS and open techniques have exhibited promising results. In a meta-analysis of outcomes following MIS and open TLIF, Khan et al noted greater improvement in back pain in those receiving MIS at 1-year follow-up.[17] Similarly, in another meta-analysis, Tian et al demonstrated greater improvement in VAS and ODI scores in those receiving MIS TLIF compared to those undergoing open TLIF.[24]

MIS TLIF has also exhibited successful outcomes in terms of stability and fusion. When utilized as a treatment for spondylolisthesis, Brodano et al demonstrated that MIS and open TLIF exhibit similar outcomes in terms of implant stability.[25] Previous studies have also noted similar rates of fusion between those receiving MIS and open TLIF.[14,25,26] Radiographically, Wang noted substantial improvements in Cobb angle, lordosis, and sagittal vertical axis at 1 year following MIS TLIF for the treatment of adult spinal deformity.[15] Similarly, other studies have noted successful correction of lumbar lordosis in the sagittal and coronal planes at 2 years following MIS TLIF.[27] These results suggest that fusions utilizing the MIS posterior approach may be efficacious in the treatment of a variety of lumbar disorders.

## References

[1] Wiltse LL, Bateman JG, Hutchinson RH, Nelson WE. The paraspinal sacrospinalis-splitting approach to the lumbar spine. J Bone Joint Surg Am. 1968; 50(5):919–926

[2] Harms J, Rolinger H. [A one-stager procedure in operative treatment of spondylolistheses: dorsal traction-reposition and anterior fusion (author's transl)]. Z Orthop Ihre Grenzgeb. 1982; 120(3):343–347

[3] Hsiang J, Yu K, He Y. Minimally invasive one-level lumbar decompression and fusion surgery with posterior instrumentation using a combination of pedicle screw fixation and transpedicular facet screw construct. Surg Neurol Int. 2013; 4:125

[4] Holly LT, Schwender JD, Rouben DP, Foley KT. Minimally invasive transforaminal lumbar interbody fusion: indications, technique, and complications. Neurosurg Focus. 2006; 20(3):E6

[5] Rouben D, Casnellie M, Ferguson M. Long-term durability of minimal invasive posterior transforaminal lumbar interbody fusion: a clinical and radiographic follow-up. J Spinal Disord Tech. 2011; 24(5):288–296

[6] Yen CP, Mosley YI, Uribe JS. Role of minimally invasive surgery for adult spinal deformity in preventing complications. Curr Rev Musculoskelet Med. 2016; 9(3):309–315

[7] Park P, Foley KT. Minimally invasive transforaminal lumbar interbody fusion with reduction of spondylolisthesis: technique and outcomes after a minimum of 2 years' follow-up. Neurosurg Focus. 2008; 25(2):E16

[8] Park Y, Ha JW, Lee YT, Oh HC, Yoo JH, Kim HB. Surgical outcomes of minimally invasive transforaminal lumbar interbody fusion for the treatment of spondylolisthesis and degenerative segmental instability. Asian Spine J. 2011; 5(4):228–236

[9] Shunwu F, Xing Z, Fengdong Z, Xiangqian F. Minimally invasive transforaminal lumbar interbody fusion for the treatment of degenerative lumbar diseases. Spine. 2010; 35(17):1615–1620

[10] Isaacs RE, Podichetty VK, Santiago P, et al. Minimally invasive microendoscopy-assisted transforaminal lumbar interbody fusion with instrumentation. J Neurosurg Spine. 2005; 3(2):98–105

[11] Mummaneni PV, Rodts GE, Jr. The mini-open transforaminal lumbar interbody fusion. Neurosurgery. 2005; 57(4) Suppl:256–261, discussion 256–261

[12] Jang JS, Lee SH. Minimally invasive transforaminal lumbar interbody fusion with ipsilateral pedicle screw and contralateral facet screw fixation. J Neurosurg Spine. 2005; 3(3):218–223

[13] Karikari IO, Isaacs RE. Minimally invasive transforaminal lumbar interbody fusion: a review of techniques and outcomes. Spine. 2010; 35(26) Suppl:S294–S301

[14] Shen X, Wang L, Zhang H, Gu X, Gu G, He S. Radiographic analysis of one-level minimally invasive transforaminal lumbar interbody fusion (MI-TLIF) with unilateral pedicle screw fixation for lumbar degenerative diseases. Clin Spine Surg. 2016; 29(1):E1–E8

[15] Wang MY. Improvement of sagittal balance and lumbar lordosis following less invasive adult spinal deformity surgery with expandable cages and percutaneous instrumentation. J Neurosurg Spine. 2013; 18(1):4–12

[16] Goldstein CL, Macwan K, Sundararajan K, Rampersaud YR. Perioperative outcomes and adverse events of minimally invasive versus open posterior lumbar fusion: meta-analysis and systematic review. J Neurosurg Spine. 2016; 24(3):416–427

[17] Khan NR, Clark AJ, Lee SL, Venable GT, Rossi NB, Foley KT. Surgical outcomes for minimally invasive vs open transforaminal lumbar interbody fusion: an updated systematic review and meta-analysis. Neurosurgery. 2015; 77(6):847–874, discussion 874

[18] Terman SW, Yee TJ, Lau D, Khan AA, La Marca F, Park P. Minimally invasive versus open transforaminal lumbar interbody fusion: comparison of clinical outcomes among obese patients. J Neurosurg Spine. 2014; 20(6):644–652

[19] Silva PS, Pereira P, Monteiro P, Silva PA, Vaz R. Learning curve and complications of minimally invasive transforaminal lumbar interbody fusion. Neurosurg Focus. 2013; 35(2):E7

[20] Nandyala SV, Fineberg SJ, Pelton M, Singh K. Minimally invasive transforaminal lumbar interbody fusion: one surgeon's learning curve. Spine J. 2014; 14(8):1460–1465

[21] Lee KH, Yeo W, Soeharno H, Yue WM. Learning curve of a complex surgical technique: minimally invasive transforaminal lumbar interbody fusion (MIS TLIF). J Spinal Disord Tech. 2014; 27(7):E234–E240

[22] Schizas C, Tzinieris N, Tsiridis E, Kosmopoulos V. Minimally invasive versus open transforaminal lumbar interbody fusion: evaluating initial experience. Int Orthop. 2009; 33(6):1683–1688

[23] Schwender JD, Holly LT, Rouben DP, Foley KT. Minimally invasive transforaminal lumbar interbody fusion (TLIF): technical feasibility and initial results. J Spinal Disord Tech. 2005; 18 Suppl:S1–S6

[24] Tian NF, Wu YS, Zhang XL, Xu HZ, Chi YL, Mao FM. Minimally invasive versus open transforaminal lumbar interbody fusion: a meta-analysis based on the current evidence. Eur Spine J. 2013; 22(8):1741–1749

[25] Brodano GB, Martikos K, Lolli F, et al. Transforaminal lumbar interbody fusion in degenerative disk disease and spondylolisthesis Grade I: minimally invasive versus open surgery. J Spinal Disord Tech. 2015; 28(10):E559–E564

[26] Kim CW, Doerr TM, Luna IY, et al. Minimally invasive transforaminal lumbar interbody fusion using expandable technology: a clinical and radiographic analysis of 50 patients. World Neurosurg. 2016; 90:228–235

[27] Dorward IG, Lenke LG, Bridwell KH, et al. Transforaminal versus anterior lumbar interbody fusion in long deformity constructs: a matched cohort analysis. Spine. 2013; 38(12):E755–E762

# 3 Posterior Retractor Systems

*Mohammed Abbas, Benjamin Khechen, Brittany E. Haws, Ankur S. Narain, Fady Hijji, Kaitlyn L. Cardinal, Jordan A. Guntin, and Kern Singh*

## 3.1 Introduction

### 3.1.1 Retractor Components

Retraction systems are composed of various components, including tubular dilators, frames, retractors, illumination devices, and camera sources. Tubular dilators are thin-walled tubular structures that are used to obtain spinal access via splitting of the muscle fascicles. In order to split the necessary muscles during surgical exposure, a series of concentric dilators are sequentially introduced.[1] Frames are metal or plastic constructs that allow for the connection and anchoring of retractor components to the surgical bed. In expandable systems, frames often contain the necessary inputs for adjustment of retractor size. The retractor apparatus can be composed of a tubular structure or bladed system. Tubular retractors, like tubular dilators, are thin walled to provide even pressure distribution on nearby musculature.[1] Due to their shape, they also provide a defined surgical corridor. Bladed retractors, unlike tubular retractors, require muscle tension to remain in position.[1] Additionally, these retractors allow for retraction in the cranial-caudal and medial-lateral planes. Various blade lengths and shapes are available to provide adequate retraction depth and orientation based on the surgical anatomy. Finally, illumination and camera systems can be fixed to the retraction frame or retractor apparatus to improve visualization in the appropriate surgical scenarios.

### 3.1.2 Types of Retraction Systems

#### Fixed versus Expandable Systems

Fixed retraction systems are those that are not adjustable in the cranial-caudal or medial-lateral planes after insertion into the target tissue. These retractors are typically composed of anodized metal and are available as tubular or bladed systems. These systems are partially or completely radiolucent, allowing for acquisition of fluoroscopic images without interference of retractor components. The benefits of a fixed tubular system include minimal muscle creep and limitation of the pressure placed on the surrounding paraspinal musculature due to consistent tube size. While fixed systems have retractors of varying lengths, complete replacement of the retractor apparatus is necessary if adjustment to sizing is required. Expandable systems, on the other hand, contain mechanisms that allow for adjustment of retractor orientation in the cranial-caudal and medial-lateral planes. As such, any repositioning required to adjust the degree of surgical exposure does not require removal of the retractor apparatus. However, muscle creep can occur and a larger retraction field is necessary, increasing the surgical dissection.

#### Pedicle-Screw–Based Systems

Pedicle-screw–based retraction systems are used in cases of degenerative disease or trauma requiring pedicle screw and rod constructs for fixation or reduction. These systems are composed of percutaneous retractor towers attached to pedicle screws at a

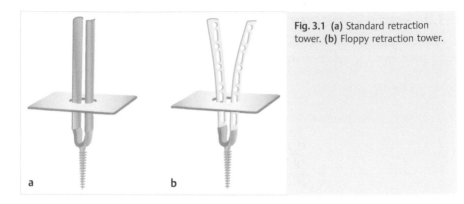

**Fig. 3.1 (a)** Standard retraction tower. **(b)** Floppy retraction tower.

fixation point. While a variety of retraction towers are currently available (▶ Fig. 3.1), the standard setup involves a simple tower that connects to the pedicle screw tulip.[2] Floppy towers utilize a soft, malleable sleeve that provides an enhanced view of the surgical field.[2] Reduction towers, currently the most utilized type, are associated with screws containing an extended internal thread which allows for greater ability to reduce deformities.[2] Overall, advantages of pedicle-screw–based systems include decreased retractor migration due to fixation of the construct to the screw, and improved visualization of anatomic landmarks. However, pedicle fracture and screw subsidence are possibilities, as distraction across the screws is often used to facilitate visualization and interbody placement.

### 3.1.3 Complications

While minimally invasive surgery decreases iatrogenic tissue trauma due to smaller exposures, utilization of tubular dilators and retractions systems is associated with a unique set of complications. Misplacement of retraction systems, regardless of the specific minimally invasive spine (MIS) procedure performed, is associated with transient neurologic deficits including numbness, paraesthesia, and pain.[3,4] The use of tubular retractors also reduces tactile feedback and the overall surgical exposure, consequently increasing the risk of iatrogenic injuries and difficulty with resolving intraoperative issues.[1]

# 3.2 Static Retractor Systems

**Table 3.1** DePuy Synthes SPOTLIGHT® Access System

| Design | | |
|---|---|---|
| **Retractor system** | **Retractor apparatus** | **Design feature** |
| Fixed | Radiolucent tube | 360° light access |

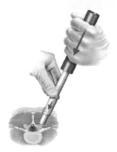 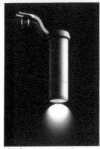

DePuy Synthes SPOTLIGHT® Spotlight Access System
illustrated upon insertion (left) and free standing (right)

| Modular aspects and variations | |
|---|---|
| **Port diameters** | **Port lengths** |
| 12, 15, 18, 21, 24 mm | 30–140 mm (10-mm increments) |

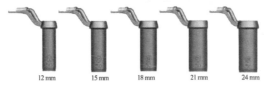

12 mm    15 mm    18 mm    21 mm    24 mm

Available diameter options for the SPOTLIGHT® Access System

| Procedures |
|---|
| MIS TLIF, MIS posterior decompression |
| Radiographs unavailable |

| Compatible devices |
|---|
| DePuy Synthes T-PAL™ Interbody Spacer System, VIPER® 2 MIS Spine System |

**Table 3.2** Medtronic METRx® II System

| Design | | |
|---|---|---|
| **Retractor system** Fixed | **Retractor apparatus** Radiolucent tube | **Design feature** Retractor available with 20° beveled tip permits docking onto the lamina |

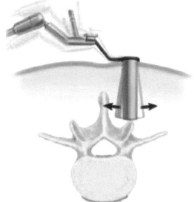

Improved positioning of the fixed tubular retractor is achieved with retractor pivoting

| Modular aspects and variations | | | | |
|---|---|---|---|---|
| **Retractor dimensions and composition** | | | | **Dilator diameter** |
| **Composition** | Beveled stainless | Straight stainless | Beveled disposable | Straight disposable | 5.3, 9.4, 12.8, 14.6 mm, 16.8–24.8 mm (2-mm increments) |
| **Widths** | 14, 16, 18, 20 mm | 22, 26 mm | 18 mm | 22, 26 mm | |
| **Lengths** | 30–90 mm (10-mm increments) | | | | |

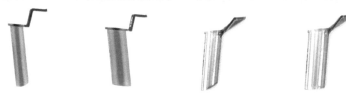

Available retractor options (left to right: beveled stainless, straight stainless, beveled disposable, straight disposable)

| Procedures |
|---|
| MIS TLIF, MIS posterior decompression |
| Radiographs unavailable |

| Compatible devices |
|---|
| Medtronic CD Horizon® Posterior Stabilization System |

**Table 3.3** RTI Surgical Clarity® MIS Port System

| Design | | |
| --- | --- | --- |
| **Retractor system**<br>Fixed | **Retractor apparatus**<br>Radiolucent tube | **Design feature**<br>Aluminum ports with dual-light access |

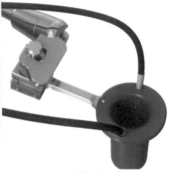

Clarity® Tube Retractor

| Modular aspects and variations | |
| --- | --- |
| **Retractor tube diameters:**<br>18, 22, and 26 mm | **Retractor tube lengths:**<br>50–120 mm (10-mm increments) |

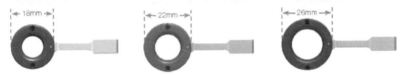

Available length options for the Clarity® Tube Retractor

| Procedures |
| --- |

MIS TLIF, MIS posterior decompression

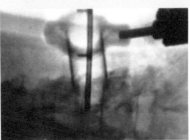

Clarity® MIS Port System on lateral fluoroscopy

| Compatible devices |
| --- |

RTI Surgical Streamline® MIS Spinal Fixation System, Bullet-tip, and T-Plus™ Interbody Cages

**Table 3.4** Zimmer Biomet Viewline™ Tube Retraction System

| Design | | |
| --- | --- | --- |
| **Retractor system**<br>Fixed | **Retractor apparatus**<br>Radiolucent tube | **Design feature**<br>Rotating accessory arm with dual-light ports |

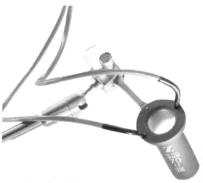

Viewline™ Tube Retractor System

| Modular aspects and variations | |
| --- | --- |
| **Retractor tube diameter**<br>18, 22, and 26 mm | **Retractor tube length**<br>40–120 mm (10-mm increments) |

  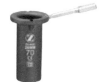

18 mm model      22 mm model      26 mm model

Available diameter options for the Viewline™ Tube Retractor System

| Procedures |
| --- |
| MIS TLIF, MIS posterior decompression |
| Radiographs unavailable |

| Compatible devices |
| --- |
| Zimmer Biomet PathFinder NXT®, minimally invasive pedicle screw system, and TM Ardis® Interbody System |

## 3.3 Expandable Retractor Systems

**Table 3.5** Alphatec Spine Illico® Posterior Thoracolumbar Retractor System

| Design | | |
|---|---|---|
| **Retractor system**<br>Expandable | **Retractor apparatus**<br>Tubular blade | **Design feature**<br>Independent blade retraction allows for improved surgical access |
| <br>Toeing Wrench | 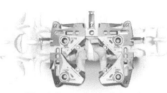<br>Illico® Expandable Retractor | <br>Distractor Tool |
| **Modular aspects and variations** | | |
| **Angulation**<br>Toeing up to 15° | **Curved blade length**<br>40–130 mm (10-mm increments) | **Distractor tool**<br>Maximum expansion of 24 × 43 mm |
| **Procedures** | | |
| MIS TLIF, MIS posterior decompression | | |
| Radiographs unavailable | | |
| **Compatible devices** | | |
| Alphatec Spine Illico® Poster Fixation System, Novel® Spinal Spacer Systems | | |

**Table 3.6** Globus Medical MARS™ Minimal Access Retractor System

| Design | | |
|---|---|---|
| **Retractor system**<br>Expandable | **Retractor apparatus**<br>Tubular blade | **Design feature**<br>Radiolucent blades provide independent retraction and angulation |

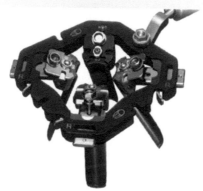

Straight medial-lateral and beveled cephalad-caudal blades support various anatomic profiles

| Modular aspects and variations | | |
|---|---|---|
| **Angulation**<br>Toeing up to 20° | **Medial-lateral and cephalad-caudal blade lengths**<br>40–120 mm (10-mm increments) | **Cannula diameters**<br>2, 5, 8, 12, 15, 18, 22 mm |

| Procedures |
|---|
| MIS TLIF, MIS posterior decompression |
| Radiographs unavailable |

| Compatible devices |
|---|
| Globus Medical REVOLVE® Stabilization System, Interbody Spacer Systems |

**Table 3.7** Medtronic MAST® Quadrant™ Retractor System

| Design | | |
| --- | --- | --- |
| **Retractor system**<br>Expandable | **Retractor apparatus**<br>Tubular blade | **Design feature**<br>Detachable retractor set in medial/lateral direction |

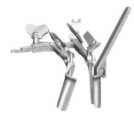 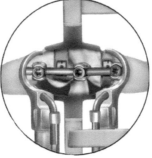 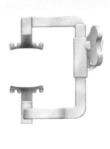

MAST® Quadrant™ Retractor utilizes 4 customizable blades to minimize tissue creep

| Modular aspects and variations | |
| --- | --- |
| **Blade length**<br>40–80 mm (10-mm increments) | **Medial/Lateral blade length**<br>50, 70, 90 mm (narrow and wide options) |

| Procedures |
| --- |
| MIS TLIF, MIS posterior decompression |
| Radiographs unavailable |

| Compatible devices |
| --- |
| Medtronic CD Horizon® Posterior Stabilization System, Interbody Spacer Systems |

**Table 3.8** SeaSpine iPassage™ MIS Retractor

| Design | | |
|---|---|---|
| Retractor system Expandable | Retractor apparatus Tubular blade | Design feature Counter retractor improves surgical access |

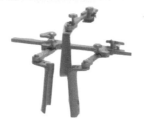

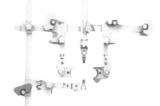

Expandable retractor allows up to 30° angulation    Counter Retractor provides 3 and 4 blade configurations

| Modular aspects and variations | | | | | |
|---|---|---|---|---|---|
| Hook length | Fan blade length | Retractor blade length | Counter retractor blade length | Dilator | |
| | | | | Composition | Diameter |
| 40–100 mm (10-mm increments) | 50–120 mm (10-mm increments) | 50–120 mm (10-mm increments) | 40–120 mm (10-mm increments) | Stainless steel | 8 mm |
| | | | | Radiolucent Aluminum | 13, 18, 22 mm |

 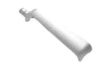  

Hook        Fan Blade    Retractor Blade (22 mm closed diameter)  Counter Retractor Blade (14 mm width)

| Procedures |
|---|
| MIS TLIF, MIS posterior decompression |
| Radiographs unavailable |

| Compatible devices |
|---|
| SeaSpine NewPort™ Posterior Stabilization System |

## 3.3.1 Flat Blade

**Table 3.9** Stryker LITe® Midline retractor

| Design | | |
|---|---|---|
| **Retractor system**<br>Expandable | **Retractor apparatus**<br>Flat blade | **Design feature**<br>Cross-cut connector prevents blade rotation while attached to blade handle |

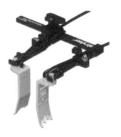
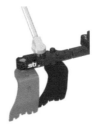

Radiolucent retractor blades provide up to 30° angulation    Two blades held per side to accommodate multi-level procedures

| Modular aspects and variations | | |
|---|---|---|
| **Angulation**<br>Toeing up to 30° | **Blade widths**<br>25 and 35 mm | **Blade lengths**<br>40–120 mm (10-mm increments) |

| Procedures |
|---|
| MIS TLIF, MIS posterior decompression |

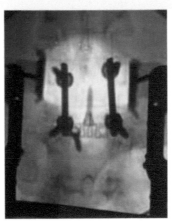

AP radiograph of the Stryker LITe® Midline Retractor

| Compatible devices |
|---|
| Stryker Supplemental Fixation System for MIS, Interbody Spacer Systems |

# 3.4 Pedicle-Screw–Based Retractor Systems

**Table 3.10** K2 M SERENGETI® Minimally Invasive Retractor System

| Design | | |
| --- | --- | --- |
| **Retractor system** Pedicle screw based | **Retractor apparatus** Floppy retraction tower | **Design feature** Polymer design allows for neuromonitoring during screw placement |

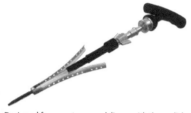

| Designed for percutaneous delivery with the pedicle screw | Provides direct visibility and access to screw heads |
| --- | --- |

| Modular aspects and variations | |
| --- | --- |
| **Dilator options** Inner and outer dilators | **Cannulated tap diameters** 4.0, 4.5–8.5 mm (1-mm increments) |

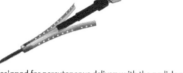

| Inner dilator | Outer dilator | Cannulated Tap |
| --- | --- | --- |

| Procedures |
| --- |
| MIS TLIF, MIS posterior decompression |
| Radiographs unavailable |

| Compatible devices |
| --- |
| K2 M EVEREST® Minimally Invasive Spinal System |

**Table 3.11** K2 M Terra Nova® Minimally Invasive Access System

### Design

| Retractor system | Retractor apparatus | Design feature |
|---|---|---|
| Pedicle screw based | Flat blade | Retractor distractor blade enables simultaneous retraction and distraction |

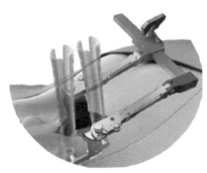

K2M Terra Nova® retractor upon insertion

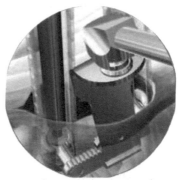

Retractor distractor blade reduces muscle creep

### Modular aspects and variations

| Medial/Lateral blades | Hook | Retractor distractor blade |
|---|---|---|
| Widths: 14 and 23 mm Lengths: 40–90 mm (10-mm increments) | Length: 40–90 mm (10-mm increments) Provides medial retraction | Widths: small, medium, and large Lengths: 50, 70, 90 mm |

### Procedures

MIS TLIF, MIS posterior decompression

Radiographs unavailable

### Compatible devices

K2 M SERENGETI®, ALEUTIAN® Interbody Spacer Systems

**Table 3.12** NuVasive MaXcess® Mas® PLIF Access System

| Design | | |
| --- | --- | --- |
| **Retractor system**<br>Pedicle screw based | **Retractor apparatus**<br>Flat blade | **Design feature**<br>Screw shank attachment and pedicle shank insertions improve stability |

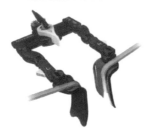 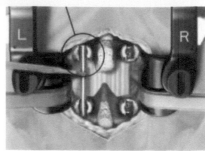

MaXcess® MAS® PLIF Access System features low-profile light cables to enhance visibility

| Modular aspects and variations | | |
| --- | --- | --- |
| **Flat blade lengths**<br>60–120 mm (10-mm increments) | **Flat blade widths**<br>Narrow, wide | **Shank diameter and length**<br>Diameters: 4.5, 5.0, 5.5, 6.5 mm<br>Lengths: 25–40 mm (5-mm increments) |

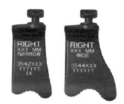 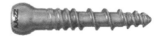

Narrow and wide flat blade options        Shank with unique threading pattern shown

| Procedures |
| --- |
| MIS PLIF, MIS posterior decompression |
| Radiographs unavailable |

| Compatible devices |
| --- |
| NuVasive CoRoent® MAS® PLIF Interbody System, Precept® MAS® PLIF Fixation System |

**Table 3.13** NuVasive MaXcess® Mas® TLIF 2 Main Access System

| Design | | |
|---|---|---|
| **Retractor system** Pedicle screw based | **Retractor apparatus** Split tube blade | **Design feature** Medial blade facilitates contralateral canal access |

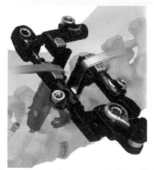 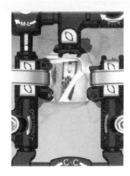

Pedicle screw based retractor sits laterally for improved direct and fluoroscopy visibility

| Modular aspects and variations | | |
|---|---|---|
| **Split tube blade lengths** 40–140 mm (10-mm increments) | **Dilator diameter** 8–20 mm (4-mm increments) | **Medial blade sizes** Extra-small, small, medium, large, and extra-large |

| Procedures |
|---|
| MIS TLIF, MIS posterior decompression |
| Radiographs unavailable |

| Compatible devices |
|---|
| NuVasive Precept® Posterior Fixation System, Reline® Modular Screw System, Interbody Spacer Systems |

# References

[1] Syed ON, Foley KT. History and evolution of minimally invasive spine surgery. In: Phillips FM, Lieberman IH, Polly Jr. DW, Wang MY, eds. Minimally Invasive Spine Surgery: Surgical Techniques and Disease Management. 1st ed. New York, New York: Springer; 2014:5

[2] Mobbs RJ, Phan K. History of retractor technologies for percutaneous pedicle screw fixation systems. Orthop Surg. 2016; 8(1):3–10

[3] Knight RQ, Schwaegler P, Hanscom D, Roh J. Direct lateral lumbar interbody fusion for degenerative conditions: early complication profile. J Spinal Disord Tech. 2009; 22(1):34–37

[4] Rodgers WB, Gerber EJ, Patterson J. Intraoperative and early postoperative complications in extreme lateral interbody fusion: an analysis of 600 cases. Spine. 2011; 36(1):26–32

# 4 Posterior Interbody Cages

*Adam B. Wiggins, Benjamin Khechen, Brittany E. Haws, Ankur S. Narain,*
*Fady Hijji, Kamran Movassaghi, Kaitlyn L. Cardinal, Jordan A. Guntin, and Kern Singh*

## 4.1 Introduction

### 4.1.1 Interbody Cage Overview

Interbody cage technology has continued to evolve since its first use in spinal fusion. Initially, autologous bone graft was utilized to induce fusion; however, this was often associated with substantial postoperative complications.[1,2,3,4,5] Interbody cages were eventually developed as a standalone construct to improve stability and distraction within the intervertebral space while also promoting bone ingrowth.[6,7] As such, interbody cages have allowed for improved fusion rates while decreasing postoperative pain, hospital length of stay, and complication rates.[8] Indications for posterior lumbar interbody cages are provided in ▶ Table 4.1.

A variety of lumbar interbody cages have been developed to maximize the implant's ability to correct deformity, provide mechanical stability, and provide the optimal environment for vertebral arthrodesis. In order to perform this, a cage must exhibit a small material volume in order to maximize the volume for bone graft.[9] Additionally, the interbody cage must exhibit a large footprint to optimize the interface between the prepared vertebral end plates and interbody cage.[10] Finally, the interbody cage should provide restoration of disk height and lordosis along with the restoration of load bearing to the anterior column.[11]

### 4.1.2 Interbody Cage Classification

#### Interbody Cage Geometry—Standard Cages

Interbody cages are classified by one of three different structures: horizontal cylinders (HCs), vertical rings (VRs), and open boxes (OBs). HCs were one of the first structures to be developed and have been considered successful in correcting deformity and providing stability.[12] However, these interbody cages are not frequently utilized in today's surgical setting.

A VR is another type of interbody cage. These interbody cages are utilized with anterior and lateral approaches to the lumbar spine. The design of VR cages was initially adapted from the design of femoral cortical rings.[13] This structure of cage has exhibited moderate ability to correct mechanical deformation. Disk height has previously been demonstrated to be maintained well with this implant, typically exhibiting an average loss of 1 mm at 1 year postoperatively.[9] Additionally, the increase in neuroforaminal area is similar to that provided by HCs.[9]

Table 4.1 Overview of surgical indications for posterior lumbar interbody cages

| Indications |
| --- |
| • Degenerative disk disease (one or two level) |
| • Spondylolisthesis (Grade 1 only) |
| • Spinal stenosis |
| • Spinal deformity |

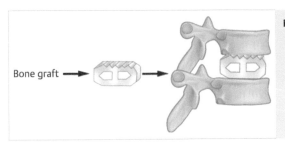

Bone graft ⟶

**Fig. 4.1** Open box interbody cage.

OB cages are the third type of geometry for interbody cages (▶ Fig. 4.1). They are one of the most frequently utilized interbody cage structures, and are often used for minimally invasive transforaminal lumbar interbody fusions (MIS TLIFs).[14] OB cages have exhibited satisfactory outcomes in correcting mechanical deformity, achieving stability, and promoting arthrodesis.[9] With appropriate surgical technique, OB cages can restore disk height and potentially increase neuroforaminal area.[9] Restoration of lumbar lordosis with OB cages has also been demonstrated to be similar to that achieved with HC cages.[14] These cages have recently been developed to exhibit a wedge shape in order to improve lordosis. OB cages have also demonstrated successful fusion rates, likely due to the sufficient volume available for bone graft and wide surface area for contact with the vertebral end plates.[9]

## Interbody Cage Geometry—Expandable Cages

Expandable interbody cages have recently been developed in attempts to overcome some of the challenges associated with minimally invasive techniques.[15] Due to the narrow surgical access corridor and anatomic positioning of minimally invasive posterior approaches, the interbody cages utilized in these techniques are often limited in size.[15,16] These smaller implants reduce the contact surface area between the vertebral end plates and the interbody cage, increasing the risk for subsidence and pseudarthrosis.[16,17,18]

Some expandable interbody cages are capable of expansion in both the medial-lateral and cranial-caudal planes. These attributes may facilitate fusion and reduce the rate of subsidence by increasing the surface area of the vertebral end plate that is in contact with the implant. However, despite these theorized benefits, there remains limited data regarding the clinical efficacy of expandable cages.[15,19]

## Interbody Cage Materials

Two predominant materials are typically utilized for interbody cages: metal and carbon fiber. Titanium is the predominant material utilized for metal cages, and polyetheretherketone (PEEK) is typically utilized in carbon fiber cages. To determine the success of a particular material for use as an interbody cage, the biologic response, biomechanical strength, and radiographic characteristics are typically assessed.

Both titanium and PEEK cages have exhibited favorable outcomes for arthrodesis and biomechanical strength. Due to the material's strength, titanium cages are thought to have increased stability and reduced micromotion when compared to PEEK cages.[9] However, PEEK cages may exhibit several advantages over titanium cages, including the avoidance of metal allergies, radiolucency, and reduced artifact on MRI.[20,21,22,23,24] These radiographic advantages allow for better analysis of arthrodesis postoperatively.

PEEK cages also exhibit moderate stiffness with some elasticity, potentially increasing fusion rates.[21] However, despite these proposed benefits, superiority of PEEK cages over titanium cages remains controversial.[25] Previous studies have demonstrated varying results, with similar fusion rates between titanium and PEEK cages.[25]

### 4.1.3 Minimally Invasive Transforaminal Lumbar Interbody Fusion

Since its introduction by Holly et al,[26] MIS TLIF has been demonstrated to reduce blood loss, postoperative pain, and length of hospital stay when compared to traditional open posterior techniques.[27,28,29,30,31,32] As such, MIS TLIF has been increasingly utilized for the treatment of degenerative lumbar disease, trauma, and deformity. However, this technique requires surgeon experience with a variety of MIS instrumentation as well as comfortability with the approach.

# 4.2 Static Carbon Fiber Interbody Cages

**Table 4.2** Alphatec Spine Novel® SD

| Design | | |
| --- | --- | --- |
| **Cage type** | **Composition** | **Design feature** |
| Static | PEEK | Multiple insertion points allow for added flexibility |

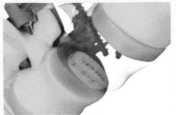

Illustration of the Novel® SD upon insertion

| Modular aspects and variations | | | |
| --- | --- | --- | --- |
| **Width** | **Length** | **Height** | **Lordotic angle** |
| 9 mm | 22, 25, 28 mm | 8–15 mm (1-mm increments) | 0° |

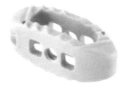 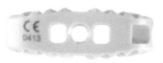

Oblique and lateral illustration of the Novel® SD

| Procedures |
| --- |
| MIS TLIF |

AP and lateral illustrations of Alphatec Novel® SD

| Supplemental fixation systems |
| --- |
| Alphatec Spine Zodiac® Polyaxial Spinal Fixation System |

**Table 4.3** Alphatec Spine Novel® Tapered TL

| Design | | |
| --- | --- | --- |
| **Cage type**<br>Static | **Composition**<br>PEEK | **Design feature**<br>Biconvex shape allows for increased endplate contact |

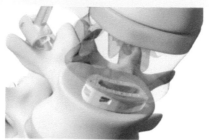

Illustration of the Novel® Tapered TL upon insertion

| Modular aspects and variations | | | |
| --- | --- | --- | --- |
| **Width**<br>10 mm | **Length**<br>24, 28, 30 mm | **Height**<br>6–15 mm (1-mm increments) | **Lordotic angle**<br>0° |

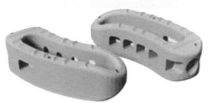

Oblique illustration of the Novel® Tapered TL

| Procedures |
| --- |
| MIS TLIF |

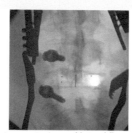 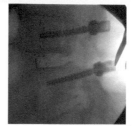

Anteroposterior and lateral fluoroscopic images of Novel® Tapered TL

| Supplemental fixation systems |
| --- |
| Alphatec Zodiac® Polyaxial Spinal Fixation System |

**Table 4.4** DePuy Synthes OPAL™ Spacer System

| Design | | |
|---|---|---|
| **Cage type** | **Composition** | **Design feature** |
| Static | PEEK | Design variations allow for two insertion options |

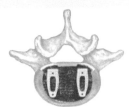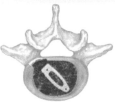

Bilateral (left) or oblique (right) placement may be utilized with OPAL™ and OPAL™ Revolve

| Modular aspects and variations | | | |
|---|---|---|---|
| **Width** | **Length** | **Height** | **Lordotic angle** |
| 9 and 10 mm | 28 and 32 mm | 7–17 mm (1-mm increments) | 0° |

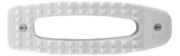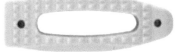

The OPAL Revolve (right) incorporates a rotational bevel for utilization of the insert and rotate technique

| Procedures |
|---|
| MIS PLIF |
| Radiographs unavailable |

| Supplemental fixation systems |
|---|
| DePuy Synthes posterior stabilization system for MIS |

**Table 4.5** DePuy Synthes T-PAL™ Interbody Spacer System

| Design | | |
|---|---|---|
| **Cage type** | **Composition** | **Design feature** |
| Static | PEEK | Incorporated TRACK technology improves implant stability |

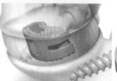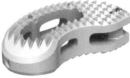

Illustration of the T-PAL Interbody Spacer System upon insertion (left) and free standing (right)

| Modular aspects and variations | | | |
|---|---|---|---|
| **Width** | **Length** | **Height** | **Lordotic angle** |
| 10 and 12 mm | 28 and 32 mm | 7–17 mm (1-mm increments) | 5° |

| Procedures |
|---|
| MIS TLIF |

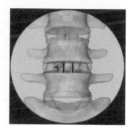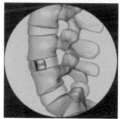

Anteroposterior and lateral fluoroscopic illustrations of T-PAL

| Supplemental fixation systems |
|---|
| DePuy Synthes posterior stabilization system for MIS |

**Table 4.6** Globus Medical SUSTAIN®-R Arch

| Design | | |
|---|---|---|
| **Cage type** | **Composition** | **Design feature** |
| Static | PEEK | Unique shape designed to follow contour of vertebral body |

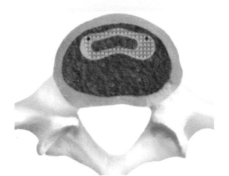

Illustration of the SUSTAIN®-R Arch upon insertion

| Modular aspects and variations | | | |
|---|---|---|---|
| **Width** | **Length** | **Height** | **Lordotic angle** |
| 10 mm | 27 and 30 mm | 7–17 mm (2-mm increments) | 0° |

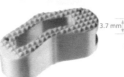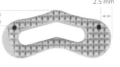

Anterior (left), oblique (middle), and superior (right) illustrations of the SUSTAIN® Arch

| Procedures |
|---|
| MIS TLIF |
| Radiographs unavailable |
| **Supplemental fixation systems** |
| Globus Medical REVOLVE® posterior stabilization system |

**Table 4.9** K2 M ALEUTIAN® AN and AN Oblique Interbody Systems

| Design | | |
|---|---|---|
| **Cage type** | **Composition** | **Design feature** |
| Static | PEEK | Bulleted nose with convex design to minimize endplate preparation |

ALEUTIAN® Anatomically-Narrow (AN) (left) and AN Oblique (right) Interbody System

| Modular aspects and variations | | | |
|---|---|---|---|
| **Width** | **Length** | **Height** | **Lordotic angle** |
| 8.5 mm | 22 and 28 mm | 6–13 mm, 15, 17 mm | 0° |
| Oblique: 8.5, 10, 12 mm | Oblique: 28 and 32 mm | Oblique: 7–15 mm | |

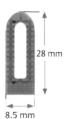 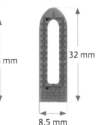 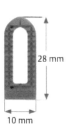 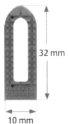 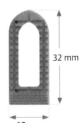

28 mm · 32 mm · 28 mm · 32 mm · 32 mm

8.5 mm · 8.5 mm · 10 mm · 10 mm · 12 mm

Available lengths for the ALEUTIAN® AN Oblique Interbody System

| Procedures |
|---|
| MIS TLIF |

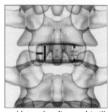 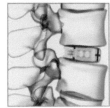

Anteroposterior and lateral radiographic illustrations of ALEUTIAN® Anatomically-Narrow (AN) Oblique

| Supplemental fixation systems |
|---|
| K2 M Terra Nova® Minimally Invasive Access System |

**Table 4.10** K2 M ALEUTIAN® TLIF 2

| Design | | |
|---|---|---|
| **Cage type** | **Composition** | **Design feature** |
| Static | PEEK | Articulating inserter allows for variable angulation from 0 to 60° in situ |

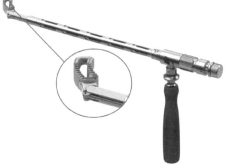 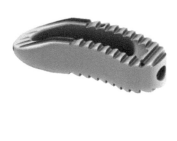

Adjustable inserter and free-standing cage shown

| Modular aspects and variations | | | |
|---|---|---|---|
| **Width** | **Length** | **Height** | **Lordotic angle** |
| 10 and 12 mm | 28, 32, 36 mm | 7–15 mm (1-mm increments) | 0 and 7° |

| Procedures |
|---|
| MIS TLIF |
| Radiographs unavailable |

| Supplemental fixation systems |
|---|
| K2 M Terra Nova® Minimally Invasive Access System |

**Table 4.11** NuVasive CoRoent® Large Contoured

| Design | | |
| --- | --- | --- |
| **Cage type** | **Composition** | **Design feature** |
| Static | PEEK | Cage curvature matches contour of vertebral body |

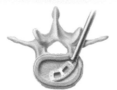 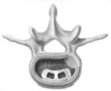

CoRoent® Large Tapered during insertion (left) and after final placement (right)

| Modular aspects and variations | | | |
| --- | --- | --- | --- |
| **Width** | **Length** | **Height** | **Lordotic angle** |
| 9 and 11 mm | 25 mm | 8–14 mm (2-mm increments) | 8° |

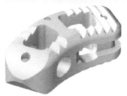 

Oblique (left) and lateral (right) illustration of the CoRoent® Large Contoured cage

| Procedures |
| --- |
| MIS TLIF, MIS LLIF |
| Radiographs unavailable |

| Supplemental fixation systems |
| --- |
| NuVasive Precept® posterior stabilization system |

**Table 4.12** NuVasive CoRoent® Large Narrow and Wide

| Design | | |
| --- | --- | --- |
| **Cage type** | **Composition** | **Design feature** |
| Static | PEEK | Designed for utilization in transforaminal, posterior, or lateral approach |

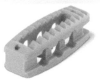 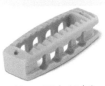

Features of the CoRoent® Large Narrow (left) and Large Wide (right) cage designs

| Modular aspects and variations | | | |
| --- | --- | --- | --- |
| **Width** | **Length** | **Height** | **Lordotic angle** |
| 9 and 11 mm | 25 and 30 mm | 8–14 mm (2-mm increments) | 0° |

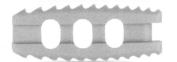 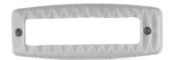

Lateral view of the CoRoent® Large Narrow (left) and superior view of the Large Wide cage design (right)

| Procedures |
| --- |
| MIS PLIF, MIS TLIF |
| Radiographs unavailable |

| Supplemental fixation systems |
| --- |
| NuVasive Precept® posterior stabilization system |

**Table 4.13** NuVasive CoRoent® Large Oblique (LO) Interbody Cage Device

| Design | | |
| --- | --- | --- |
| Cage type | Composition | Design feature |
| Static | PEEK | Designed specifically for oblique placement |

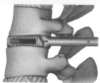 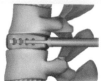

CoRoent® LO placement utilizes the Insert (left) and Rotate (right) technique

| Modular aspects and variations | | | |
| --- | --- | --- | --- |
| Width | Length | Height | Lordotic angle |
| 10 mm | 25, 30, 35, 40 mm | 8, 10, 12, 14 mm | 5° |

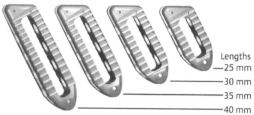

Lengths
—25 mm
—30 mm
—35 mm
—40 mm

Available Length for the CoRoent® LO

| Procedures |
| --- |
| MIS TLIF, MIS LLIF |

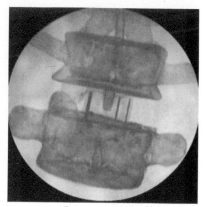 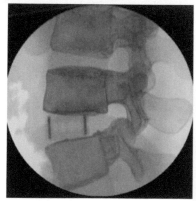

Anteroposterior and lateral fluoroscopic images of the CoRoent® LO cage

| Supplemental fixation systems |
| --- |
| NuVasive Precept® posterior stabilization system |

**Table 4.14** NuVasive CoRoent® Large Tapered Interbody Cage Device

| Design | | |
|---|---|---|
| **Cage type** | **Composition** | **Design feature** |
| Static | PEEK | Anatomical lordotic design induces proper sagittal balance |

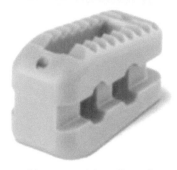

Features of the CoRoent® Large Tapered cage design

| Modular aspects and variations | | | |
|---|---|---|---|
| **Width** | **Length** | **Height** | **Lordotic angle** |
| 9 mm | 20 mm | 8–14 mm (2-mm increments) | 8 and 15° |

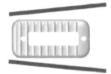 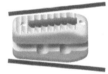 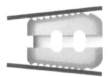

CoRoent® Large Tapered cage placement utilizes the patented Insert and Rotate techniques (left to right)

| Procedures |
|---|
| MIS PLIF, MIS LLIF |
| Radiographs unavailable |

| Supplemental fixation systems |
|---|
| NuVasive Precept® posterior stabilization system |

**Table 4.17** RTI surgical T-Plus™

| Design | | |
| --- | --- | --- |
| **Cage type** | **Composition** | **Design feature** |
| Static | PEEK | Cage curvature matches contour of vertebral body |

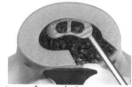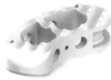

Features of cage design upon insertion (left) and free standing (right)

| Modular aspects and variations | | | |
| --- | --- | --- | --- |
| **Width** | **Length** | **Height** | **Lordotic angle** |
| 10 mm | 27 and 36 mm | 7–15 mm (1-mm increments) | 0 and 6° |

| Procedures |
| --- |
| MIS TLIF |

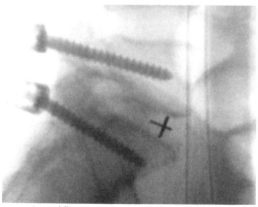

Lateral fluoroscopic image of the T-Plus™ cage

| Supplemental fixation systems |
| --- |
| RTI Surgical Streamline® MIS spinal fixation system |

**Table 4.18** SeaSpine Hollywood™

| Design | | |
|---|---|---|
| **Cage type** | **Composition** | **Design feature** |
| Static | PEEK | Cage curvature matches that of vertebral end plate |

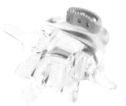 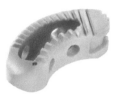

Oblique views of the Hollywood™ cage

| Modular aspects and variations | | | |
|---|---|---|---|
| **Width** | **Length** | **Height** | **Lordotic angle** |
| 11 mm | 27 mm | 7–18 mm (1-mm increments) | 8° |

| Procedures |
|---|
| MIS TLIF |

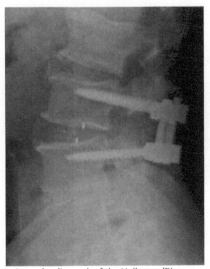

Lateral radiograph of the Hollywood™ cage

| Supplemental fixation systems |
|---|
| SeaSpine posterior stabilization systems for MIS |

# 4.3 Static Metal Interbody Cages

Table 4.21 Alphatec Spine Novel® SD

| Design | | |
|---|---|---|
| **Cage type** | **Composition** | **Design feature** |
| Static | Titanium | Multiple insertion points for added procedural flexibility |

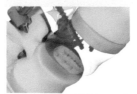 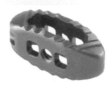

Illustration of the Novel® SD upon insertion (left) and free standing (right)

| Modular aspects and variations | | | |
|---|---|---|---|
| **Width** | **Length** | **Height** | **Lordotic angle** |
| 9 mm | 22, 25, 28 mm | 8–15 mm (1-mm increments) | 0° |

| Procedures |
|---|
| MIS TLIF |
| Radiographs unavailable |

| Supplemental fixation systems |
|---|
| Alphatec Spine Zodiac® Polyaxial Spinal Fixation System |

**Table 4.22** DePuy Synthes Concorde® Bullet Ti

| Design | | |
|---|---|---|
| **Cage type** | **Composition** | **Design feature** |
| Static | Titanium | Angled nose facilitates easier cage insertion |

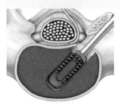 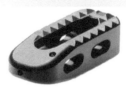

Illustration of the Concorde® Bullet upon insertion (left) and free-standing oblique view (right)

| Modular aspects and variations | | | |
|---|---|---|---|
| **Width** | **Length** | **Height** | **Lordotic angle** |
| 9 and 11 mm | 23 and 27 mm | 7–13 mm (1-mm increments) | 0 and 5° |

| Procedures |
|---|
| MIS TLIF |

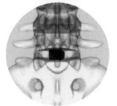 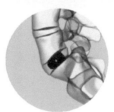

Anteroposterior and lateral illustrations of Concorde® Bullet

| Supplemental fixation systems |
|---|
| DePuy Synthes supplemental fixation systems for MIS |

**Table 4.23** Globus Medical SUSTAIN® Arch

| Design | | |
|---|---|---|
| **Cage type** | **Composition** | **Design feature** |
| Static | Titanium | Shape designed to follow contour of vertebral body |

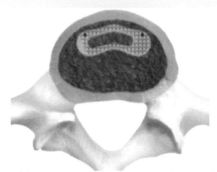

Illustration of the SUSTAIN® Arch upon insertion (PEEK model shown)

| Modular aspects and variations | | | |
|---|---|---|---|
| **Width** | **Length** | **Height** | **Lordotic angle** |
| 10 mm | 27 mm | 7–17 mm (2-mm increments) | 0° |

 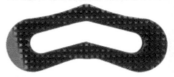

Anterior (left) and superior (right) illustration of the SUSTAIN® Arch

| Procedures |
|---|
| MIS TLIF |
| Radiographs unavailable |

| Supplemental fixation systems |
|---|
| Globus Medical REVOLVE® posterior stabilization system for MIS |

**Table 4.24** Globus Medical SUSTAIN® Small and Small Narrow

| Design | | |
| --- | --- | --- |
| **Cage type** | **Composition** | **Design feature** |
| Static | Titanium | Large axial window for graft material |

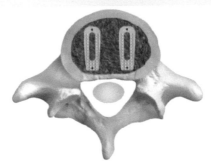

SUSTAIN® Small and Small Narrow are designed for bilateral placement (PEEK model shown)

| Modular aspects and variations | | | |
| --- | --- | --- | --- |
| **Width** | **Length** | **Height** | **Lordotic angle** |
| 8 and 10 mm | 22 mm | 7–17 mm (2 mm increments) | 7° |

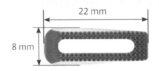 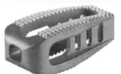 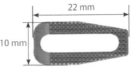

Oblique illustration of the SUSTAIN® Small (middle) and available footprint options

| Procedures |
| --- |
| MIS TLIF |

Radiographs unavailable

| Supplemental fixation systems |
| --- |

Globus Medical REVOLVE® posterior stabilization system for MIS

**Table 4.25** K2 M CASCADIA™ AN

| Design | | |
|---|---|---|
| **Cage type** | **Composition** | **Design feature** |
| Static | Titanium | Porous titanium technology for bony integration of the implant |

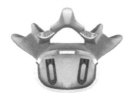 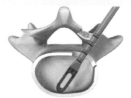

Bilateral (left) or oblique (right) placement may be utilized with CASCADIA™

| Modular aspects and variations | | | |
|---|---|---|---|
| **Width** | **Length** | **Height** | **Lordotic angle** |
| 10 mm | 22, 28, 32 mm | 7–15 mm (1-mm increments) | 0° |

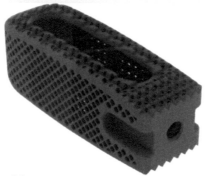

Illustration of the CASCADIA™ design, noting the convex cage design

**Table 4.25** (*Continued*) K2 M CASCADIA™ AN

| Procedures |
| --- |
| MIS PLIF, MIS TLIF |

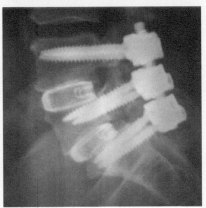

Lateral radiograph of the CASCADIA™ AN cage

| Supplemental fixation systems |
| --- |
| K2 M Terra Nova® Minimally Invasive Access System |

**Table 4.26** K2 M CASCADIA™ TL

| Design | | |
| --- | --- | --- |
| **Cage type** | **Composition** | **Design feature** |
| Static | Titanium | Porous titanium technology allows for bony integration of the implant |

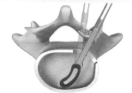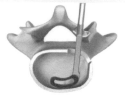

Cage design during insertion (left) and following placement (right)

| Modular aspects and variations | | | |
| --- | --- | --- | --- |
| **Width** | **Length** | **Height** | **Lordotic angle** |
| 10 mm | 28 and 32 mm | 7–15 mm | 7° |

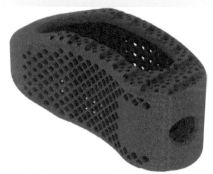

Illustration of the CASCADIA™ TL, noting the bullet-nose design

| Procedures |
| --- |
| MIS TLIF |

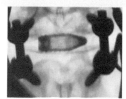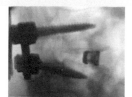

Anteroposterior and lateral radiographs of the CASCADIA™ TL cage

| Supplemental fixation systems |
| --- |
| K2 M Terra Nova® Minimally Invasive Access System |

**Table 4.27** Stryker Tritanium® PL

| Design | | |
| --- | --- | --- |
| **Cage type** | **Composition** | **Design feature** |
| Static | Titanium | Smooth exterior to prevent abrasion, porous interior to enhance fusion |

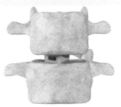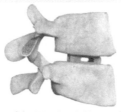

Anterior/Posterior and lateral illustration of the Tritanium® PL upon insertion

| Modular aspects and variations | | | |
| --- | --- | --- | --- |
| **Width** | **Length** | **Height** | **Lordotic angle** |
| 9 and 11 mm | 23 mm | 7–14 mm (1-mm increments) | 0 and 6° |

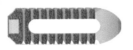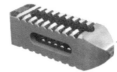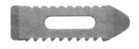

Superior, oblique, and lateral illustrations of the Tritanium® PL

| Procedures |
| --- |
| MIS PLIF |

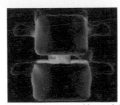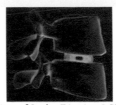

Anteroposterior and lateral illustrations of Stryker Tritanium® PL

| Supplemental fixation systems |
| --- |
| Stryker Xia CT, Radius, Trio, Techtonix, UniVise®, or ES2® posterior stabilization systems |

**Table 4.28** Zimmer Biomet TM Ardis® Interbody System

| Design | | |
| --- | --- | --- |
| **Cage type** | **Composition** | **Design feature** |
| Static | Porous tantalum | Trabecular metal material enhances bony integration |

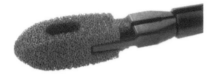

Illustration of the TM Ardis® Interbody System cage design

| Modular aspects and variations | | | |
| --- | --- | --- | --- |
| **Width** | **Length** | **Height** | **Lordotic angle** |
| 9 and 11 mm | 26, 30, 34 mm | 8–14 mm (1-mm increments), 16 mm | 0° |

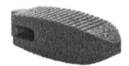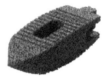

Oblique illustrations of the TM Ardis® Interbody System cage design

| Procedures |
| --- |
| MIS PLIF, MIS TLIF |

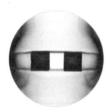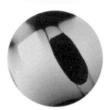

Anteroposterior and lateral illustrations of TM Ardis® Interbody System

| Supplemental fixation systems |
| --- |
| Zimmer Biomet Pathfinder NXT® posterior stabilization systems |

# 4.4 Static Mixed Composition Interbody Cages

**Table 4.29** Alphatec Spine Battalion™ PC

| Design | | |
|---|---|---|
| **Cage type** | **Composition** | **Design feature** |
| Static | PEEK with TPS | Unique inserter 180° locking mechanism aids in implantation, and convex design improves cage fit |

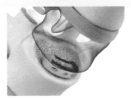 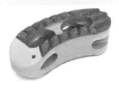

Illustration of the Alphatec Spine Battalion™ PC upon insertion (left) and free standing (right)

| Modular aspects and variations | | | |
|---|---|---|---|
| **Width** | **Length** | **Height** | **Lordotic angle** |
| 10 mm | 25, 30, 35 mm | 7–15 mm (1-mm increments) | 0° |

| Procedures |
|---|
| MIS TLIF |

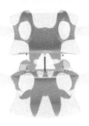 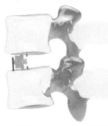

Anteroposterior and lateral illustrations of Alphatec Spine Battalion™ PC

| Supplemental fixation systems |
|---|
| Alphatec Spine Zodiac® Spinal Fixation System |

**Table 4.30** Alphatec Spine Battalion™ PS

| Design | | |
| --- | --- | --- |
| **Cage type** | **Composition** | **Design feature** |
| Static | PEEK with TPS | Designed for bilateral or oblique placement |

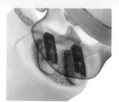 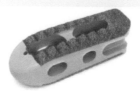

Illustration of the Alphatec Spine Battalion™ PS upon insertion (left) and free standing (right)

| Modular aspects and variations | | | |
| --- | --- | --- | --- |
| **Width** | **Length** | **Height** | **Lordotic angle** |
| 10 mm | 25, 30, 35 mm | 7–15 mm (1-mm increments) | 0° |

| Procedures |
| --- |
| MIS TLIF |

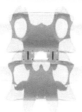 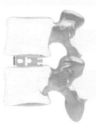

Anteroposterior and lateral illustrations of bilateral Alphatec Spine Battalion™ PS

| Supplemental fixation systems |
| --- |
| Alphatec Spine Zodiac® Spinal Fixation System |

**Table 4.31** Globus Medical SUSTAIN®-O TPS

| Design | | |
|---|---|---|
| **Cage type** | **Composition** | **Design feature** |
| Static | PEEK with TPS | Surfaces feature directional teeth to resist expulsion |

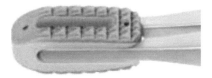

The anterior tapered edge and rounded corners enhance control during insertion and placement

| Modular aspects and variations | | | |
|---|---|---|---|
| **Width** | **Length** | **Height** | **Lordotic angle** |
| 8, 10, 12 mm | 22, 26, 30 mm | 8–13 mm (1-mm increments), 15, 17 mm | 7° |

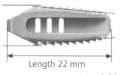 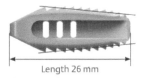 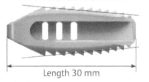

| Length 22 mm | Length 26 mm | Length 30 mm |
|---|---|---|

Available length options for SUSTAIN®-O TPS Interbody Cage

| Procedures |
|---|
| MIS TLIF |
| Radiographs unavailable |

| Supplemental fixation systems |
|---|
| Globus Medical REVOLVE® posterior stabilization system for MIS |

**Table 4.32** Medtronic Capstone PTC™

| Design | | |
| --- | --- | --- |
| Cage type | Composition | Design feature |
| Static | PEEK with TPS | Large central graft chamber for enhanced fusion potential |

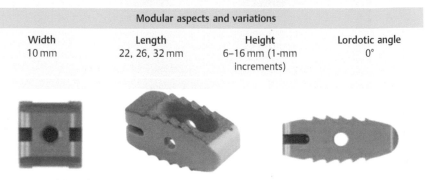

Bilateral or oblique placement may be utilized with the Capstone PTC™

| Modular aspects and variations | | | |
| --- | --- | --- | --- |
| Width | Length | Height | Lordotic angle |
| 10 mm | 22, 26, 32 mm | 6–16 mm (1-mm increments) | 0° |

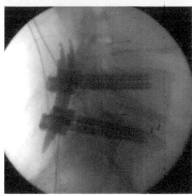

Posterior (left), oblique (middle), and lateral (right) illustration of the Capstone PTC™ cage design

| Procedures |
| --- |
| MIS PLIF, MIS TLIF |

Lateral fluoroscopic image of Medtronic Capstone PTC™

| Supplemental fixation systems |
| --- |
| Medtronic supplemental fixation systems for MIS |

**Table 4.33** SeaSpine Hollywood™ NanoMetalene®

| Design | | |
| --- | --- | --- |
| **Cage type** | **Composition** | **Design feature** |
| Static | PEEK with NanoMetalene® | NanoMetalene® coating maintains radiolucency |

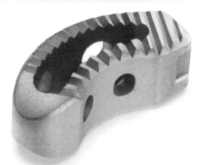

Illustration of the Hollywood™ NanoMetalene® cage design

| Modular aspects and variations | | | |
| --- | --- | --- | --- |
| **Width** | **Length** | **Height** | **Lordotic angle** |
| 11 mm | 27 mm | 7–18 mm (1-mm increments) | 8° |

| Procedures |
| --- |
| MIS TLIF |

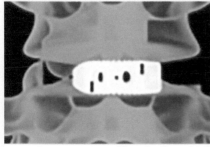 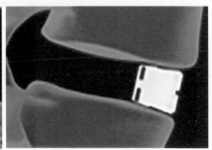

Anteroposterior and lateral radiographic illustrations of Hollywood™ NanoMetalene®

| Supplemental fixation systems |
| --- |
| SeaSpine NewPort™ posterior stabilization system for MIS |

**Table 4.34** SeaSpine Ventura™ NanoMetalene®

| Design | | |
| --- | --- | --- |
| **Cage type** | **Composition** | **Design feature** |
| Static | PEEK with NanoMetalene® | NanoMetalene® coating maintains radiolucency |

 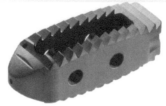 

Anterior (left), oblique (middle), and posterior (right) illustrations of the Ventura™ NanoMetalene® cage design

| Modular aspects and variations | | | |
| --- | --- | --- | --- |
| **Width** | **Length** | **Height** | **Lordotic angle** |
| 9 and 11 mm | 28 and 32 mm | 7–13 mm (1-mm increments), 15, 17 mm | 0° |

| Procedures |
| --- |
| MIS TLIF |

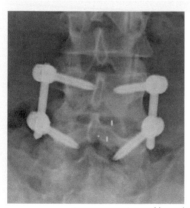 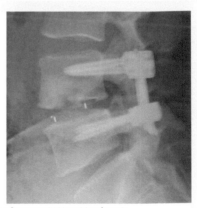

Anteroposterior and lateral radiographs of Ventura™ NanoMetalene®

| Supplemental fixation systems |
| --- |
| SeaSpine NewPort™ posterior stabilization system |

# 4.5 Static Allograft Interbody Cages

**Table 4.35** Globus Medical FORGE® Oblique Allograft Spacer

| Design | | |
| --- | --- | --- |
| **Cage type** | **Composition** | **Design feature** |
| Static | Cortical bone | Recessed holder slots minimize interference during insertion |

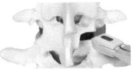 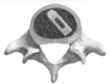

Illustration of the Globus Medical FORGE® upon insertion (left) and following placement (right)

| Modular aspects and variations | | | |
| --- | --- | --- | --- |
| **Width** | **Length** | **Height** | **Lordotic angle** |
| 10 mm | 26 and 30 mm | 7–13 mm (1-mm increments), 15, 17 mm | 7° |

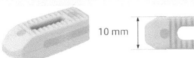

Oblique (left) and superior (right) illustration of the Globus Medical FORGE® allograft spacer

| Procedures |
| --- |
| MIS TLIF |

Radiographs unavailable

| Supplemental fixation systems |
| --- |

Globus Medical REVOLVE® posterior stabilization system for MIS

**Table 4.36** NuVasive Triad Allograft Spacer

| Design | | |
|---|---|---|
| **Cage type**<br>Static | **Composition**<br>Cortical bone allograft | **Design feature**<br>Saline storage solution eases allograft preparation |

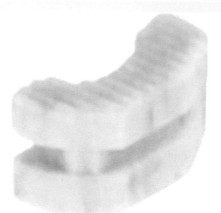

Oblique illustration of the NuVasive Triad allograft spacer

| Modular aspects and variations | | | |
|---|---|---|---|
| **Width**<br>9 and 11 mm | **Length**<br>20 and 25 mm | **Height**<br>8, 10, 12, 14 mm | **Lordotic angle**<br>0° |

| Procedures |
|---|
| MIS TLIF |
| Radiographs unavailable |

| Supplemental fixation systems |
|---|
| NuVasive Precept® posterior stabilization system |

**Table 4.37** Zimmer Biomet Fortis PLIF Allograft Interbody Spacer

| Design | | |
|---|---|---|
| **Cage type** | **Composition** | **Design feature** |
| Static | Cortical/Cancellous allograft | Prominent superior and inferior ridges resist migration |

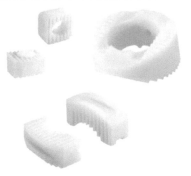

Illustration of the Fortis collection of allograft spacers

| Modular aspects and variations | | | |
|---|---|---|---|
| **Width** | **Length** | **Height** | **Lordotic angle** |
| 10 mm | 20 mm, 24 mm | 8–14 mm (2-mm increments) | 0° |

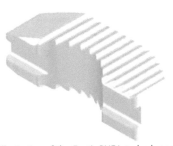

Illustration of the Fortis PLIF interbody spacer

| Procedures |
|---|
| MIS PLIF |
| Radiographs unavailable |

| Supplemental fixation systems |
|---|
| Zimmer Biomet PathFinder NXT™ posterior stabilization system |

# 4.6 Expandable Interbody Cages

Table 4.38 Benvenue Medical Luna™ 3D

| Design | | |
|---|---|---|
| **Cage type** Expandable | **Composition** PEEK | **Design feature** The Luna™ 3D is inserted through a unique cannula in two stages |

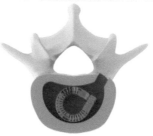

Illustration of the Luna™ 3D upon insertion

| Modular aspects and variations | | |
|---|---|---|
| **Initial heights** 5–7.5 mm (0.5-mm increments) | **Expansion ranges** 8–13 mm (1-mm increments) | **Lordotic angle** 0° |

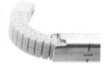 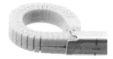 

Top and bottom components are initially delivered (left, center), followed by the middle component (right)

| Procedures |
|---|
| MIS PLIF |

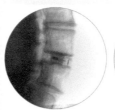 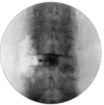

Anteroposterior and lateral fluoroscopic images of Luna™ 3D

| Supplemental fixation systems |
|---|
| Benvenue Medical posterior stabilization systems for MIS |

**Table 4.39** Globus Medical ALTERA™ Interbody Cage

| Design | | |
| --- | --- | --- |
| **Cage type**<br>Expandable | **Composition**<br>PEEK with titanium | **Design feature**<br>Protrusions increase endplate grip and resist expulsion |

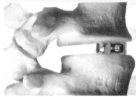
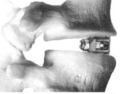

Cage design upon initial insertion (left) and following expansion (right)

| Modular aspects and variations | | |
| --- | --- | --- |
| **Expansion ranges**<br>8–12, 9–13, 10–14, 12–16 mm | **Footprint options**<br>10 × 26, 10 × 31, 10 × 36 mm | **Lordotic angle**<br>8 and 15° |

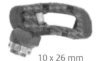
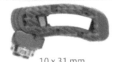
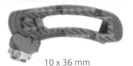

10 x 26 mm          10 x 31 mm          10 x 36 mm

Available footprints for the ALTERA™ interbody cage

| Procedures |
| --- |
| MIS TLIF |

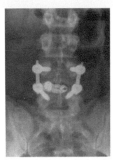
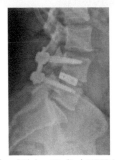

Anteroposterior and lateral radiographs of Globus Medical ALTERA™

| Supplemental fixation systems |
| --- |
| Globus Medical REVOLVE® posterior stabilization system for MIS |

**Table 4.40** Globus Medical CALIBER® Interbody Cage

| Design | | |
| --- | --- | --- |
| **Cage type**<br>Expandable | **Composition**<br>PEEK with titanium | **Design feature**<br>Adjustable lordotic angle model<br>for a customized fit |

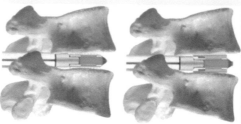

Cage design upon initial insertion (left) and following expansion (right)

| Modular aspects and variations | | |
| --- | --- | --- |
| **Footprint options**<br>10 × 22, 10 × 26, 10 × 30 mm<br>12 × 22, 12 × 26, 12 × 30 mm | **Expansion ranges**<br>7–12, 8–13, 9–14, 10–15,<br>11–16, 12–17 mm | **Lordotic angle**<br>4°, 12°, 15° and adjustable<br>model |

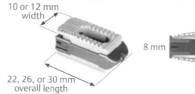
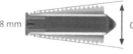
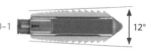

Available footprints (left), with adjustable lordotic angle model (middle) and adjustable model (right)

| Procedures |
| --- |
| MIS TLIF |
| Radiographs unavailable |

| Supplemental fixation systems |
| --- |
| Globus Medical REVOLVE® posterior stabilization system for MIS |

**Table 4.41** Globus Medical LATIS® Interbody Cage

| Design | | |
| --- | --- | --- |
| **Cage type** | **Composition** | **Design feature** |
| Expandable | Titanium | Utilizes a single instrument for insertion, expansion, and graft delivery |

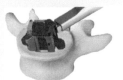 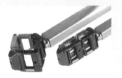

Fully expanded, LATIS® provides a large graft chamber

| Modular aspects and variations | | |
| --- | --- | --- |
| **Footprint options** | **Height** | **Lordotic angle** |
| 10 × 32, 10 × 37 mm | 7–15 mm (1-mm increments), 17 mm | 0° |

0%
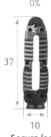
37
10

50%
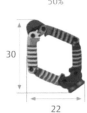
30
22

100%
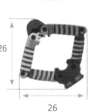
26
26

Secure locking at incremental expansion ranges allows for a custom footprint (10 × 37mm model shown)

| Procedures |
| --- |
| MIS TLIF |
| Radiographs unavailable |

| Supplemental fixation systems |
| --- |
| Globus Medical REVOLOVE® posterior stabilization system for MIS |

**Table 4.42** Medtronic Elevate™

| Design | | |
|---|---|---|
| **Cage type**<br>Expandable | **Composition**<br>PEEK with titanium | **Design feature**<br>0° and adjustable lordotic options for customization |

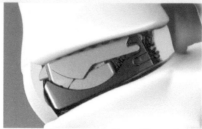

Illustration of the Medtronic Elevate™ upon insertion

| Modular aspects and variations | | | |
|---|---|---|---|
| **Width**<br>10 mm | **Length**<br>23, 28, 32 mm | **Expansion ranges**<br>8–12, 9–13, 10–14, 11–15 mm | **Lordotic angle**<br>Adjustable 8–15° |

 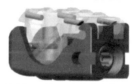 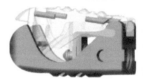

Posterior (left), oblique (middle), and lateral (right) illustration of the Medtronic Elevate™ cage design

**Table 4.42** (*Continued*) Medtronic Elevate™

| Procedures |
| --- |
| MIS PLIF, MIS TLIF, MIS MIDLF |

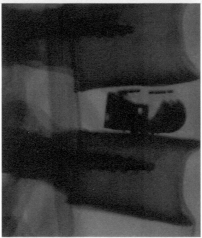

Lateral fluoroscopic image of Medtronic Elevate™

| Supplemental fixation systems |
| --- |
| Medtronic supplemental stabilization system for MIS |

# References

[1] Glassman SD, Dimar JR, Carreon LY, Campbell MJ, Puno RM, Johnson JR. Initial fusion rates with recombinant human bone morphogenetic protein-2/compression resistant matrix and a hydroxyapatite and tricalcium phosphate/collagen carrier in posterolateral spinal fusion. Spine. 2005; 30(15):1694–1698

[2] Boden SD. Overview of the biology of lumbar spine fusion and principles for selecting a bone graft substitute. Spine. 2002; 27(16) Suppl 1:S26–S31

[3] Ludwig SC, Kowalski JM, Boden SD. Osteoinductive bone graft substitutes. Eur Spine J. 2000; 9 Suppl 1:S119–S125

[4] Lind M, Bünger C. Factors stimulating bone formation. Eur Spine J. 2001; 10 Suppl 2:S102–S109

[5] Vaccaro AR, Sharan AD, Tuan RS, et al. The use of biologic materials in spinal fusion. Orthopedics. 2001; 24(2):191–197, quiz 198–199

[6] DeBowes RM, Grant BD, Bagby GW, Gallina AM, Sande RD, Ratzlaff MH. Cervical vertebral interbody fusion in the horse: a comparative study of bovine xenografts and autografts supported by stainless steel baskets. Am J Vet Res. 1984; 45(1):191–199

[7] Ray CD. Threaded titanium cages for lumbar interbody fusions. Spine. 1997; 22(6):667–679, discussion 679–680

[8] Dimar JR, Glassman SD, Burkus KJ, Carreon LY. Clinical outcomes and fusion success at 2 years of single-level instrumented posterolateral fusions with recombinant human bone morphogenetic protein-2/compression resistant matrix versus iliac crest bone graft. Spine. 2006; 31(22):2534–2539, discussion 2540

[9] Weiner BK, Fraser RD. Spine update lumbar interbody cages. Spine. 1998; 23(5):634–640

[10] Steffen T, Tsantrizos A, Fruth I, Aebi M. Cages: designs and concepts. Eur Spine J. 2000; 9 Suppl 1:S89–S94

[11] Tsantrizos A, Andreou A, Aebi M, Steffen T. Biomechanical stability of five stand-alone anterior lumbar interbody fusion constructs. Eur Spine J. 2000; 9(1):14–22

[12] Bagby GW. Arthrodesis by the distraction-compression method using a stainless steel implant. Orthopedics. 1988; 11(6):931–934

[13] Kozak JA, O'Brien JP. Simultaneous combined anterior and posterior fusion. An independent analysis of a treatment for the disabled low-back pain patient. Spine. 1990; 15(4):322–328

[14] Brantigan JW, Steffee AD, Geiger JM. A carbon fiber implant to aid interbody lumbar fusion. Mechanical testing. Spine. 1991; 16(6) Suppl:S277–S282

[15] Cannestra AF, Peterson MD, Parker SR, Roush TF, Bundy JV, Turner AW. MIS expandable interbody spacers: a literature review and biomechanical comparison of an expandable MIS TLIF with conventional TLIF and ALIF. Spine. 2016; 41 Suppl 8:S44–S49

[16] Tan JS, Bailey CS, Dvorak MF, Fisher CG, Oxland TR. Interbody device shape and size are important to strengthen the vertebra-implant interface. Spine. 2005; 30(6):638–644

[17] Oxland TR, Grant JP, Dvorak MF, Fisher CG. Effects of endplate removal on the structural properties of the lower lumbar vertebral bodies. Spine. 2003; 28(8):771–777

[18] Lowe TG, Hashim S, Wilson LA, et al. A biomechanical study of regional endplate strength and cage morphology as it relates to structural interbody support. Spine. 2004; 29(21):2389–2394

[19] Kim CW, Doerr TM, Luna IY, et al. Minimally invasive transforaminal lumbar interbody fusion using expandable technology: a clinical and radiographic analysis of 50 patients. World Neurosurg. 2016; 90:228–235

[20] Tanida S, Fujibayashi S, Otsuki B, et al. Vertebral endplate cyst as a predictor of nonunion after lumbar interbody fusion: comparison of titanium and polyetheretherketone cages. Spine. 2016; 41(20):E1216–E1222

[21] Vadapalli S, Sairyo K, Goel VK, et al. Biomechanical rationale for using polyetheretherketone (PEEK) spacers for lumbar interbody fusion - a finite element study. Spine. 2006; 31(26):E992–E998

[22] Toth JM, Wang M, Estes BT, Scifert JL, Seim HB, III, Turner AS. Polyetheretherketone as a biomaterial for spinal applications. Biomaterials. 2006; 27(3):324–334

[23] Ferguson SJ, Visser JM, Polikeit A. The long-term mechanical integrity of non-reinforced PEEK-OPTIMA polymer for demanding spinal applications: experimental and finite-element analysis. Eur Spine J. 2006; 15(2):149–156

[24] Cabraja M, Oezdemir S, Koeppen D, Kroppenstedt S. Anterior cervical discectomy and fusion: comparison of titanium and polyetheretherketone cages. BMC Musculoskelet Disord. 2012; 13:172

[25] Nemoto O, Asazuma T, Yato Y, Imabayashi H, Yasuoka H, Fujikawa A. Comparison of fusion rates following transforaminal lumbar interbody fusion using polyetheretherketone cages or titanium cages with transpedicular instrumentation. Eur Spine J. 2014; 23(10):2150–2155

[26] Holly LT, Schwender JD, Rouben DP, Foley KT. Minimally invasive transforaminal lumbar interbody fusion: indications, technique, and complications. Neurosurg Focus. 2006; 20(3):E6

[27] Foley KT, Holly LT, Schwender JD. Minimally invasive lumbar fusion. Spine. 2003; 28(15) Suppl:S26–S35

[28] Isaacs RE, Podichetty VK, Santiago P, et al. Minimally invasive microendoscopy-assisted transforaminal lumbar interbody fusion with instrumentation. J Neurosurg Spine. 2005; 3(2):98–105

[29] Mummaneni PV, Rodts GE, Jr. The mini-open transforaminal lumbar interbody fusion. Neurosurgery. 2005; 57(4) Suppl:256–261, discussion 256–261

[30] Jang JS, Lee SH. Minimally invasive transforaminal lumbar interbody fusion with ipsilateral pedicle screw and contralateral facet screw fixation. J Neurosurg Spine. 2005; 3(3):218–223

[31] Schwender JD, Holly LT, Rouben DP, Foley KT. Minimally invasive transforaminal lumbar interbody fusion (TLIF): technical feasibility and initial results. J Spinal Disord Tech. 2005; 18 Suppl:S1–S6

[32] Shunwu F, Xing Z, Fengdong Z, Xiangqian F. Minimally invasive transforaminal lumbar interbody fusion for the treatment of degenerative lumbar diseases. Spine. 2010; 35(17):1615–1620

# 5 Percutaneous Pedicle Screw Systems

*Simon P. Lalehzarian, Benjamin Khechen, Brittany E. Haws, Jordan A. Guntin, Kaitlyn L. Cardinal, and Kern Singh*

## 5.1 Introduction

Pedicle screws evolved from the original facet screw technique to improve spinal internal fixation while maintaining vertebral range of motion.[1] With the use of plates or rods, pedicle screws can provide load sharing between vertebrae, improving overall fixation and preventing vertebral collapse.[2,3] Multiple methods have been developed to improve pedicle screw fixation strength, such as improving insertional torque, cross-linking adjacent screws, and triangulating the insertion of the screw.[2] In minimally invasive spine surgery, percutaneous pedicle screw insertion techniques are utilized. The pedicle screw is oriented approximately 30° from vertical to allow for accurate pedicle insertion in addition to improving screw pull-out strength (▸ Fig. 5.1).[4] Surgical indications for percutaneous pedicle screws are described in ▸ Table 5.1.

### 5.1.1 Pedicle Screw Components

A pedicle screw is composed of a head, or tulip, neck, and shaft. The head is where the rods are placed to interconnect consecutive screws. Screw heads can be fixed (monoaxial) or can allow motion at the shaft–head interface (polyaxial). While polyaxial screws

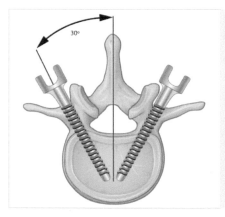

**Fig. 5.1** Illustration of the target trajectory for pedicle screw placement.

**Table 5.1** Surgical indications for percutaneous pedicle screws

**Indications**

- Posterior approach spinal fusion
- Thoracolumbar procedures
- Degenerative disk disease
- Spondylolisthesis
- Spinal fracture/dislocation
- Spinal stenosis
- Spinal deformity

allow for easier rod insertion, they are also associated with failure at lower loads and greater rates of screw-head slippage than monoaxial screws.[5,6] Monoplanar screws have also been introduced, which allow for motion in the axial plane while maintaining rigidity in the sagittal plane.[7,8] In percutaneous pedicle screw placement, tulip extensions provide a corridor through which the screw head can be accessed from outside of the patient.[9] These extensions can either be removable or fixed with a break-off tab for removal. Tulip extensions are traditionally rigid, but can be malleable or lie flat against the skin for increased visualization. Additionally, some systems have capabilities for reduction or deformity correction. However, literature comparing the efficacy between tulip extension designs is limited and thus, choice of system is largely based on surgeon preference.

The screw shaft can be conical or cylindrical in shape. Conical screws have previously been associated with greater insertional torque and bending performance.[10,11] However, concerns exist regarding the pullout strength of conical screws when backed out 360°.[12] The shaft also contains the threads of the screw. The height and size of the thread crests determine the inner and outer diameter of the screw shaft (▶ Fig. 5.2). The outer diameter of the screw shaft has been identified as a major determinant of pullout strength, while the inner diameter is reported to determine the fatigue strength.[12,13] Different thread options are available, including double lead and dual thread screws which facilitate faster insertion and increase insertional torque.[12,14] The distance between the crest of each thread is called the pitch, and this measurement is also thought to be crucial in determining pullout strength of the screw. When screw pullout occurs, the bone in between the crests of each thread is often fractured. As such, the amount of bone in between the threads and the quality of bone can directly impact screw strength.

Percutaneous pedicle screw placement is performed by using Kirschner wires to determine accurate trajectory under fluoroscopic guidance. Cannulated screws are then introduced over the guidewire. The hollow core of cannulated screws has raised concerns over increased risk for screw breakage as compared to solid screws. Studies have suggested that cannulated screws exhibit decreased mechanical strength, stiffness, and axial failure loads when compared to solid screws of similar diameters.[15,16] As such, it is recommended that cannulated cores not exceed 2.0 mm in diameter.[17] However,

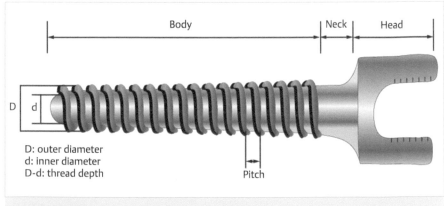

Body | Neck | Head

D
d
D: outer diameter
d: inner diameter
D-d: thread depth
Pitch

**Fig. 5.2** Illustration of the components of a pedicle screw.

previous reports have determined that cannulated conical screws are able to maintain the bending performance of solid screws, suggesting that conical designs are preferred for cannulated screw placement.[18,19] Newer designs have been proposed that use an additional pin to fill the cannulated core in an attempt to recreate the structural stability of the solid screw. However, this design has not been determined to improve the bending performance of cannulated screws.[18]

## 5.1.2 Pedicle Screw Constructs

Multiple constructs have been developed to improve pedicle screw strength and efficacy. These devices are often classified as rigid, semirigid, or dynamic stabilization systems. Variations in the materials utilized to create interconnecting rods and screws are what determine the type of stabilization system. Lumbar fusion with rigid posterior instrumentation is thought to increase fusion rates in cases of degenerative spinal disorders.[20] However, these rigid systems have also previously been associated with some undesirable outcomes, including loss of lumbar lordosis, stress-shielding, adjacent segment degeneration, and fatigue fractures.[21,22] Semirigid and dynamic systems were developed as a method of enhancing load sharing as opposed to stress shielding. Additionally, dynamic stabilization is thought to reduce susceptibility to adjacent segment degeneration.[23,24,25] Despite the theoretical benefits of less rigid systems in the setting of lumbar spinal fixation, superiority over rigid systems has been difficult to elucidate.[20,26]

## 5.1.3 Complications

The complications associated with pedicle screws and the accuracy of pedicle screw placement have been reviewed thoroughly throughout the literature.[27] Inaccurate screw placement is a common concern, particularly with percutaneous techniques, as visualization is limited. Medially misplaced screws can result in impingement or displacement of traversing nerve roots or dural tears. Additionally, screws angled cephalad with superior facet joint violation have been suggested to increase the risk of early failure or adjacent segment disease due to increased intrapedicular bending movements.[28,29] While superior facet violation has been suggested to occur in approximately 18% of pedicle screw placements, similar rates have been demonstrated for both open and percutaneous techniques.[30]

## 5.2 Percutaneous Pedicle Screw Systems

**Table 5.2** Alphatec Spine Illico® MIS Posterior Fixation System

| Design | |
| --- | --- |
| **Set screws specifications**<br>Standard T25 drive mechanism<br>Designed to limit cross-threading | **Reduction capabilities**<br>Zodiac® cannulated high-top screws may be<br>used to facilitate reduction |

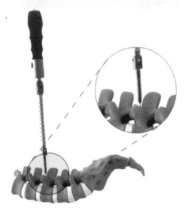 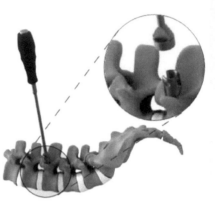

Polyaxial screw insertion with screwdriver (left) and realignment with head positioner (right)

| Modular aspects and variations | | | |
| --- | --- | --- | --- |
| **Screw diameters**<br>5.5, 6.5, 7.5 mm | **Screw lengths**<br>35–55 mm<br>(5-mm increments) | **Rod type**<br>Precontoured<br>Straight | **Rod lengths**<br>30–100 mm (5-mm<br>increments)<br>200 mm |

| Procedures |
| --- |
| MIS TLIF, MIS posterior decompression |

Radiographs unavailable

**Table 5.3** DePuy Synthes VIPER® MIS Spine System

| Design | |
| --- | --- |
| **Set screws specifications**<br>Standard T25 drive mechanism | **Reduction capabilities**<br>X-Tab reduction screw: up to 7-mm reduction |

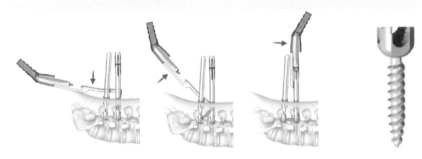

Rod placement with angled rod holder (left) and free-standing polyaxial screw (right)

| Modular aspects and variations | | | |
| --- | --- | --- | --- |
| **Screw diameter** | **Screw lengths** | **Rod type** | **Rod lengths** |
| 4.35, 5.0, 6.0, 7.0, 7.5, 8.0, 9.0 mm | 30–55 mm (5-mm increments) | Straight | 35, 40–120 (10-mm increments), 150, 200, 300, 400, 600 mm |
| | | Kyphosed | 35, 40–120 (10-mm increments), 150, 200, 300 mm |
| | | Lordosed | 30–90 (5-mm increments), 100, 110, 120, 150, 200 mm |

| Procedures |
| --- |
| MIS TLIF, MIS posterior decompression |

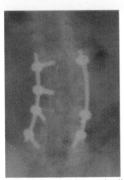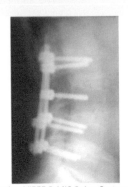

Anteroposterior and lateral radiographs illustrating VIPER® MIS Spine System placement

**Table 5.4** Globus Medical CREO MIS™ Posterior Stabilization System

| Design | |
| --- | --- |
| **Set screw specifications**<br>Threaded locking cap with 8.0 mm of torque for final tightening | **Reduction capability**<br>Reduction options include 10 and 30 mm |

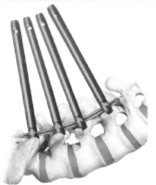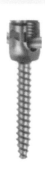

Creo MIS™ Posterior Stabilization System offers minimal screw sleeve interference during reduction

| Modular aspects and variations | | | |
| --- | --- | --- | --- |
| **Screw diameters**<br>4.5–8.5 (1-mm increments), 5.0 mm | **Screw lengths**<br>20–120 mm | **Rod diameters**<br>5.5 and 6 mm | **Rod lengths**<br>30–150 mm (5-mm increments)<br>160–300 mm (10-mm increments) |

| Procedures |
| --- |
| MIS TLIF, MIS posterior decompression |

Radiographs unavailable

**Table 5.5** K2 M EVEREST® Minimally Invasive Spinal System

| Design | |
| --- | --- |
| **Set screws specifications** | **Reduction capabilities** |
| Modified square thread design | Multiple reduction constructs up to 20 mm |
| Designed to facilitate easy introduction and limit cross-threading | |

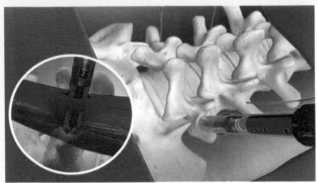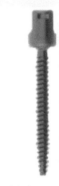

Polyaxial screw insertion with SERENGETI® retractor (left) and free-standing cannulated screw (right)

| Modular aspects and variations | | | |
| --- | --- | --- | --- |
| **Screw diameters** | **Screw lengths** | **Rode type** | **Rod lengths** |
| 5.5–8.5 mm | 35–55 mm (5-mm increments) | Contoured | 5.5 and 6 mm |

| Procedures |
| --- |
| MIS TLIF, MIS posterior decompression |

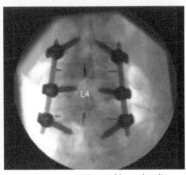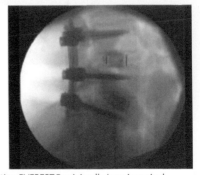

Anteroposterior and lateral radiographs illustrating EVEREST® minimally invasive spinal system placement

**Table 5.6** Medtronic CD Horizon® Longitude® II Multilevel Percutaneous Fixation System

| Design | |
| --- | --- |
| **Set screws specifications** Tulip designed to reduce anatomical impact | **Reduction capabilities** Staged reduction technique allows for accurate screw placement |

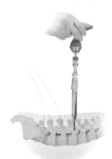 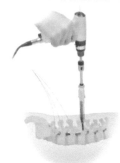 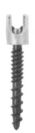

Multiaxial screw insertion using screw extender assembly with guidewire (left, center) and free-standing multiaxial screw (right)

| Modular aspects and variations | | | |
| --- | --- | --- | --- |
| **Screw diameters** | **Screw lengths** | **Rod type** | **Rod lengths** |
| 4.5 mm | 30, 35, 40 mm | Prebent | 30–80 mm (5-mm |
| 5.5 mm | 30–50 mm (5-mm | Straight | increments) |
| 6.5 and 7.5 mm | increments) | | 70–260 mm (10-mm |
| 8.5, 9.5, 10.5 mm | 35–55 mm (5-mm | | increments) |
| | increments) | | |
| | 90, 100, 110 mm | | |

| Procedures |
| --- |
| MIS TLIF, MIS posterior decompression |

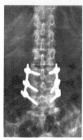 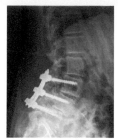

Anteroposterior and lateral radiographs illustrating Medtronic Longitude® II Percutaneous Fixation System placement

**Table 5.7** Medtronic CD Horizon® Solera® Spinal System

| Design | |
| --- | --- |
| **Set screw specifications**<br>Reverse angle thread locking mechanism | **Reduction capability**<br>Multiple reduction devices available for different diameter rods |

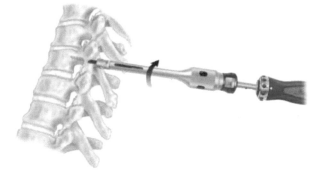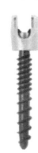

Screw placement using multiaxial screw lock sleeve driver (left)
and free-standing multiaxial screw (right)

**Modular aspects and variations**

| Screw diameter | Screw lengths | Rod type | Rod lengths |
| --- | --- | --- | --- |
| 4–6 mm (0.5-mm increments), 6.5–9.5 mm (1.0-mm increments) | 20–60 mm (5-mm increments) | Pre-bent<br>Straight | 30–120 mm (5-mm increments)<br>500, 600 mm |

| Procedures |
| --- |

MIS TLIF, MIS posterior decompression

Radiographs unavailable

**Table 5.8** Medtronic CD Horizon® Solera® Voyager Spinal System

| Design | |
|---|---|
| **Set screws specifications** | **Reduction capabilities** |
| Utilizes tulip design to reduce anatomical impact | Break-off section of tab extenders allows for 13.8 mm of reduction |

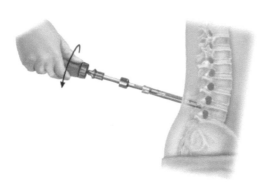 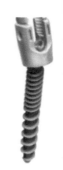

Multiaxial screw insertion using screw extender assembly with guidewire (left) and free-standing multiaxial screw (right)

| Modular aspects and variations | | | |
|---|---|---|---|
| **Screw diameters** | **Screw lengths** | **Rod type** | **Rod lengths** |
| 4.5 mm | 35, 40, 45 mm | Percutaneous | 30–90 mm (5-mm increments) |
| 5.5 mm | 35–50 mm (5-mm increments) | Capped | 30–80 mm (5-mm increments) |
| 6.5 and 7.5 mm | 35–55 mm (5-mm increments) | | |

| Procedures |
|---|
| MIS TLIF, MIS posterior decompression |
| Radiographs unavailable |

**Table 5.9** NuVasive Reline® Posterior Fixation System

| Design | |
|---|---|
| **Set screw specifications** | **Reduction capability** |
| Helical flange and metric thread locking mechanisms | Reduction capabilities ranging from 9 to 50 mm |

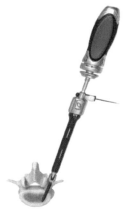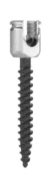

Screw insertion using polyaxial screwdriver (left) and free-standing polyaxial screw (right)

| Modular aspects and variations | | | |
|---|---|---|---|
| **Screw diameters** | **Screw lengths** | **Rod type** | **Rod lengths** |
| 5.5, 6.5, 7.5, 8.5 mm | 35–55 mm (5-mm increments) | Lordotic Straight | 25–100 (5-mm increments), 110, 120, 140, 160, 300 mm |

| Procedures |
|---|
| MIS TLIF, MIS posterior decompression |
| Radiographs unavailable |

**Table 5.10** NuVasive SpheRx® DBR III Spinal System

| Design | |
| --- | --- |
| **Set screw specifications** | **Reduction capability** |
| Designed to limit cross-threading and allow "instrument-free" compression | Reduction can be achieved using DBR III counter-torque/reduction sleeve, reduction T-handle, and reducer extension |

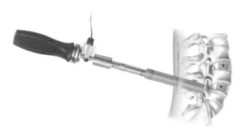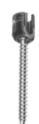

Polyaxial screw insertion using SpheRx® DBR III screwdriver with standard DBR III guide (left) and free-standing polyaxial screw (right)

| Modular aspects and variations | | | |
| --- | --- | --- | --- |
| **Screw diameter** | **Screw lengths** | **Rod type** | **Rod lengths** |
| 5.5, 6.5, 7.5 mm | 30–55 mm (5-mm increments) | Pre-bent<br>Pre-bent dual ball<br>Straight dual ball | 20–110 (5-mm increments), 120, 130, 140, 150 mm<br>25–70 mm (2.5-mm increments)<br>17.5, 20, 22.5, 72.5, 75, 77.5, 80 mm |

| Procedures |
| --- |
| MIS TLIF, MIS posterior decompression |

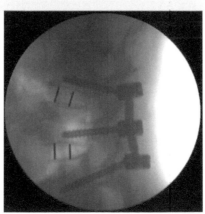

Lateral fluoroscopic image of NuVasive SpheRx® DBR III Spinal System placement

**Table 5.11** RTI Surgical Streamline® MIS Spinal Fixation System

| Design | |
|---|---|
| **Set screws specifications** | **Reduction capabilities** |
| Standard T25 drive mechanism | Simple rod inserter: up to 15-mm reduction |
| Designed to limit cross-threading | Rod reducers: up to 30-mm reduction |

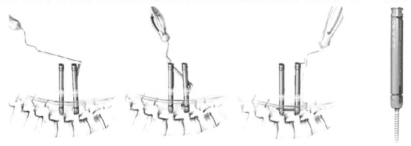

Rod placement with fixed rod holder and free-standing conical screw with extension sleeve

| Modular aspects and variations | | | |
|---|---|---|---|
| **Screw diameter** | **Screw lengths** | **Rod type** | **Rod lengths** |
| 4.5–8.5 mm | 30–55 mm | Pre-bent | 35–80 mm (5-mm |
| (1-mm increments) | (5-mm increments) | Straight | increments) |
| | | Long | 90–150 mm (10-mm |
| | | | increments) |
| | | | 160–250 mm (10-mm |
| | | | increments) |

| Procedures |
|---|
| MIS TLIF, MIS posterior decompression |

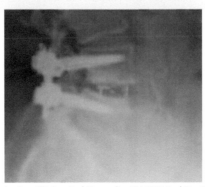

Lateral radiograph illustrating RTI Surgical Streamline® MIS Spinal Fixation System placement

**Table 5.12** Zimmer Biomet PathFinder NXT™ Pedicle Screw Fixation System

| Design | |
|---|---|
| **Set screws specifications**<br>Standard T25 drive mechanism<br>Designed to limit cross-threading | **Reduction capability**<br>Reduction forceps: up to 10-mm reduction<br>Power knob reducer: up to 30-mm reduction |

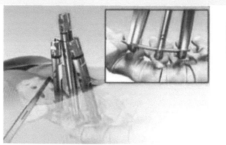

Percutaneous pre-bent rod placement and insertion and free-standing polyaxial screw

| Modular aspects and variations | | | |
|---|---|---|---|
| **Screw diameters**<br>4.5–7.5 mm (1-mm<br>increments) | **Screw lengths**<br>30–60 mm (5-mm<br>increments) | **Rod type**<br>Pre-bent<br>Straight | **Rod lengths**<br>30–100 mm (5-mm<br>increments)<br>100–240 mm (20-mm<br>increments) |

| Procedures |
|---|
| MIS TLIF, MIS posterior decompression |

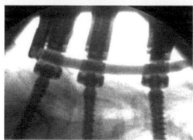

Lateral fluoroscopic image of PathFinder NXT™ Pedicle Screw Fixation System placement

# References

[1] Boucher HH. A method of spinal fusion. J Bone Joint Surg Br. 1959; 41-B(2):248–259

[2] Gaines RW, Jr. The use of pedicle-screw internal fixation for the operative treatment of spinal disorders. J Bone Joint Surg Am. 2000; 82(10):1458–1476

[3] Gaines RW, Jr, Carson WL, Satterlee CC, Groh GI. Experimental evaluation of seven different spinal fracture internal fixation devices using nonfailure stability testing. The load-sharing and unstable-mechanism concepts. Spine. 1991; 16(8):902–909

[4] Mobbs RJ, Sivabalan P, Li J. Technique, challenges and indications for percutaneous pedicle screw fixation. J Clin Neurosci. 2011; 18(6):741–749

 [5] Fogel GR, Reitman CA, Liu W, Esses SI. Physical characteristics of polyaxial-headed pedicle screws and biomechanical comparison of load with their failure. Spine. 2003; 28(5):470–473

 [6] Serhan H, Hammerberg K, O'Neil M, Sturm P, Mardjetko S, Crawford A. Intraoperative techniques to reduce the potential of set-screw loosening in long spinal constructs: a static and fatigue biomechanical investigation. J Spinal Disord Tech. 2010; 23(7):e31–e36

 [7] Schroerlucke SR, Steklov N, Mundis GM, Jr, Marino JF, Akbarnia BA, Eastlack RK. How does a novel monoplanar pedicle screw perform biomechanically relative to monoaxial and polyaxial designs? Clin Orthop Relat Res. 2014; 472(9):2826–2832

 [8] Ye B, Yan M, Zhu H, et al. Novel screw head design of pedicle screw for reducing the correction loss in the patients with thoracolumbar vertebral fractures: a biomechanical study. Spine. 2017; 42(7):E379–E384

 [9] Mobbs RJ, Phan K. History of retractor technologies for percutaneous pedicle screw fixation systems. Orthop Surg. 2016; 8(1):3–10

[10] Kwok AW, Finkelstein JA, Woodside T, Hearn TC, Hu RW. Insertional torque and pull-out strengths of conical and cylindrical pedicle screws in cadaveric bone. Spine. 1996; 21(21):2429–2434

[11] Chao CK, Hsu CC, Wang JL, Lin J. Increasing bending strength and pullout strength in conical pedicle screws: biomechanical tests and finite element analyses. J Spinal Disord Tech. 2008; 21(2):130–138

[12] Cho W, Cho SK, Wu C. The biomechanics of pedicle screw-based instrumentation. J Bone Joint Surg Br. 2010; 92(8):1061–1065

[13] Bianco RJ, Arnoux PJ, Wagnac E, Mac-Thiong JM, Aubin CÉ. Minimizing pedicle screw pullout risks: a detailed biomechanical analysis of screw design and placement. Clin Spine Surg. 2017; 30(3):E226–E232

[14] Mummaneni PV, Haddock SM, Liebschner MA, Keaveny TM, Rosenberg WS. Biomechanical evaluation of a double-threaded pedicle screw in elderly vertebrae. J Spinal Disord Tech. 2002; 15(1):64–68

[15] Bava E, Charlton T, Thordarson D. Ankle fracture syndesmosis fixation and management: the current practice of orthopedic surgeons. Am J Orthop. 2010; 39(5):242–246

[16] Yang SW, Kuo SM, Chang SJ, et al. Biomechanical comparison of axial load between cannulated locking screws and noncannulated cortical locking screws. Orthopedics. 2013; 36(10):e1316–e1321

[17] Chang CM, Lai YS, Cheng CK. Effect of different inner core diameters on structural strength of cannulated pedicle screws under various lumbar spine movements. Biomed Eng Online. 2017; 16(1):105

[18] Shih KS, Hsu CC, Hou SM, Yu SC, Liaw CK. Comparison of the bending performance of solid and cannulated spinal pedicle screws using finite element analyses and biomechanical tests. Med Eng Phys. 2015; 37(9):879–884

[19] Reese K, Litsky A, Kaeding C, Pedroza A, Shah N. Cannulated screw fixation of Jones fractures: a clinical and biomechanical study. Am J Sports Med. 2004; 32(7):1736–1742

[20] Korovessis P, Papazisis Z, Koureas G, Lambiris E. Rigid, semirigid versus dynamic instrumentation for degenerative lumbar spinal stenosis: a correlative radiological and clinical analysis of short-term results. Spine. 2004; 29(7):735–742

[21] Shono Y, Kaneda K, Abumi K, McAfee PC, Cunningham BW. Stability of posterior spinal instrumentation and its effects on adjacent motion segments in the lumbosacral spine. Spine. 1998; 23(14):1550–1558

[22] Zindrick MR, Wiltse LL, Widell EH, et al. A biomechanical study of intrapeduncular screw fixation in the lumbosacral spine. Clin Orthop Relat Res. 1986(203):99–112

[23] Stoll TM, Dubois G, Schwarzenbach O. The dynamic neutralization system for the spine: a multi-center study of a novel non-fusion system. Eur Spine J. 2002; 11 Suppl 2:S170–S178

[24] Putzier M, Schneider SV, Funk JF, Tohtz SW, Perka C. The surgical treatment of the lumbar disc prolapse: nucleotomy with additional transpedicular dynamic stabilization versus nucleotomy alone. Spine. 2005; 30(5):E109–E114

[25] Schnake KJ, Schaeren S, Jeanneret B. Dynamic stabilization in addition to decompression for lumbar spinal stenosis with degenerative spondylolisthesis. Spine. 2006; 31(4):442–449

[26] Fokter SK, Strahovnik A. Dynamic versus rigid stabilization for the treatment of disc degeneration in the lumbar spine. Evid Based Spine Care J. 2011; 2(3):25–31

[27] Lonstein JE, Denis F, Perra JH, Pinto MR, Smith MD, Winter RB. Complications associated with pedicle screws. J Bone Joint Surg Am. 1999; 81(11):1519–1528

[28] Youssef JA, McKinley TO, Yerby SA, McLain RF. Characteristics of pedicle screw loading. Effect of sagittal insertion angle on intrapedicular bending moments. Spine. 1999; 24(11):1077–1081

[29] Cardoso MJ, Dmitriev AE, Helgeson M, Lehman RA, Kuklo TR, Rosner MK. Does superior-segment facet violation or laminectomy destabilize the adjacent level in lumbar transpedicular fixation? An in vitro human cadaveric assessment. Spine. 2008; 33(26):2868–2873

[30] Wang L, Wang Y, Yu B, Li Z, Li Y. Comparison of cranial facet joint violation rate between percutaneous and open pedicle screw placement: a systematic review and meta-analysis. Medicine (Baltimore). 2015; 94(5):e504

# 6 Cortical Screw Systems

*Simon P. Lalehzarian, Benjamin Khechen, Brittany E. Haws, Kaitlyn L. Cardinal, Jordan A. Guntin, Sravisht Iyer, and Kern Singh*

## 6.1 Introduction

The posterior approach for cortical screw fixation is described in Chapter 3 Posterior Retractor Systems. Posterior screw fixation with a cortical trajectory was initially described by Santoni et al in 2009.[1] Cortical screws were developed with the intention of maximizing cortical bone purchase, which has proven advantageous in conditions such as osteoporosis where trabecular bone may not have adequate density to achieve stable fixation.[2] Regarding placement, the cortical screw start point is located at the junction of the superior articular process and pars interarticularis.[3] Utilization of this start point allows for intraoperative preservation of muscle attachments, and possible reduced postoperative pain.[3,4,5] The trajectory of cortical screws is lateral and cephalad from the start point.[6] This trajectory allows for placement of the screw within the cortical bone of the pedicle, rather than entering the trabecular bone of the vertebral body as is the case with pedicle screws. Minimally invasive cortical screw placement can be utilized during midline lumbar fusion (MIDLF), which involves a posterior midline approach and microsurgical laminectomy, followed by cortical screw fixation.[7,8] This technique reduces the risk of neural injury due to the medial to lateral and caudal to cephalad trajectory of the cortical screw (▶ Fig. 6.1).[7] Additionally, MIDLF provides for decompression and fusion through the same surgical corridor, further reducing tissue dissection and retraction.[7]

### 6.1.1 Components

The dimensions of cortical screws necessarily differ from those of pedicle screws. Cortical screws have a denser thread, larger minor diameter, and a smaller bite than traditional cancellous pedicle screws (▶ Fig. 6.2).[9] The denser thread and amount of depth per rotation aid insertion into harder cortical bone. Cortical screws are also shorter

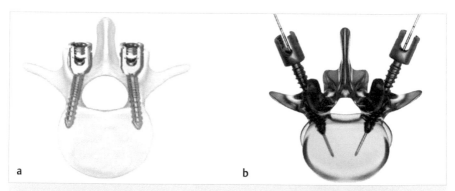

a                                      b

**Fig. 6.1** Screw trajectories for **(a)** cortical screws (Arsenal CBx) and **(b)** pedicle screws (Illico MIS posterior fixation).

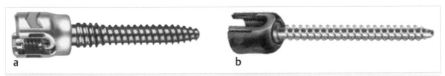

**Fig. 6.2** Dimension differences between **(a)** cortical (CREO MCS, Globus Medical) and **(b)** pedicle screws (SpheRx DBR III, NuVasive, Inc.).

than pedicle screws, so as not to violate the pedicle borders or enter the trabecular bone of the vertebral body. Similar to pedicle screws, the heads of cortical screws contain articulating tulips that allow for percutaneous placement of rods to promote stable fixation of two vertebral levels.

## 6.1.2 Efficacy and Complications

The effectiveness of cortical screw fixation has been extensively studied from a biomechanical perspective. Many biomechanical studies utilizing cadaveric spine constructs have demonstrated that cortical screws are at least equivalent to pedicle screws in regard to bone purchase.[2,9,10,11,12,13] Regarding strength, multiple studies have indicated that cortical screws have a superior strength profile compared to pedicle screws. Cortical screws have demonstrated increased resistance to craniocaudal toggling forces, greater insertional torque, and a greater pullout load required before screw failure occurs. The increased strength of cortical screws is attributed to the cortical, rather than trabecular, trajectory of placement within the pedicle.

The study of peri- and postoperative outcomes after cortical screw fixation is an emerging topic in the literature, with recent data providing promising results. Studies have demonstrated reduced surgical morbidity with the use of cortical screws compared to pedicle screws.[3,4,5,8] Cortical screw use has been associated with shorter incision lengths, shorter operative times, reduced intraoperative blood loss, and reduced inpatient postoperative pain. These improvements have been attributed to minimization of soft-tissue distraction and retention afforded by the more medial screw start point. Longer-term postoperative outcomes, however, have been mixed.[3,5] Some studies have demonstrated similar pain, functional status, and fusion rates at 12 months postoperatively in cohorts receiving either cortical or pedicle screws.[5] Other studies have noted an increased pain profile in cortical screw cohorts at 6 to 8 months postoperatively.[3] Further prospective, controlled studies are required to better elucidate the long-term clinical and radiographic efficacy of cortical versus pedicle screws.

Complications encountered when utilizing cortical screw fixation significantly overlap with reported complications associated with pedicle screw fixation.[14,15] Most complications of cortical screw trajectory have been reported in small case series or small prospective studies. Reported complications in those studies have included hardware failure, screw loosening, pars fracture, pedicle fracture, durotomy, and pseudarthrosis. A unique complication involving difficulty of rod placement due to screw head misalignment has also been reported in cortical screw cohorts.[8] While the majority of studies indicate a low complication rate with the utilization of cortical screws, few studies have compared the rates of these complications in pedicle versus cortical screw groups. Larger case series and prospective studies are required for a meaningful comparison of complication rate between the two primary options for screw fixation.

## 6.2 Cortical Screw Systems

**Table 6.1** Alphatec Spine Arsenal™ CBx Cortical Bone Fixation System

| Design | |
| --- | --- |
| **Set screw specifications**<br>Uses a T27 drive mechanism<br>Utilizes tulip design to reduce anatomical impact | **Reduction capabilities**<br>Reduction capabilities range from 9 to 30 mm |

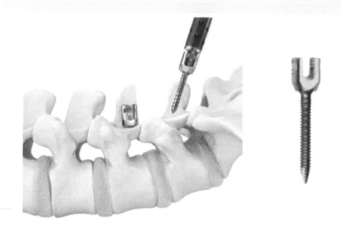

Cortical screw insertion (left), with cortical screw (center right), and corticocancellous screw (far right)

| Modular aspects and variations | |
| --- | --- |
| **Screw diameter**<br>4–6.5 mm (0.5-mm increments) | **Rod type**<br>Precontoured, straight |

| Procedures |
| --- |
| MIS TLIF, MIS MIDLF |
| Radiographs unavailable |

| Supplemental fixation systems |
| --- |
| Alphatec Spine Illico® Posterior Stabilization System |

**Table 6.2** DePuy Synthes Spine VIPER® Cortical Fix Screw System

| Design |
| --- |

**Set screw specifications**
Tulip design to reduce anatomical impact

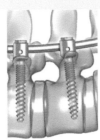 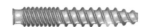

Screw insertion with rod, set screws, and tulip head design (left) and cortical fix screw with dual
thread lead (right)

| Modular aspects and variations | |
| --- | --- |
| **Screw diameters**<br>5–9 mm (1-mm increments) | **Screw lengths**<br>30–55 mm (5-mm increments) |

| Procedures |
| --- |

MIS TLIF, MIS MIDLF

Radiographs unavailable

| Supplemental fixation systems |
| --- |

DePuy Synthes EXPEDIUM® Spine System, VIPER® System

**Table 6.3** Globus Medical CREO MCS™ Midline Cortical Stabilization System

| Design | |
| --- | --- |
| **Set screw specifications** | **Reduction capabilities** |
| Nonthreaded locking cap technology prevents cross-threading | 5 reduction options for up to 20 mm of reduction |

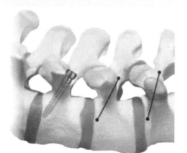 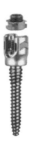 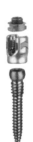

CREO MCS™ screw insertion and cortical trajectories (left), preassembled screw (middle), and modular screw (right)

| Modular aspects and variations | |
| --- | --- |
| **Screw diameter** | **Rod diameters** |
| 7 mm | 4.75, 5.5, 6.35 mm |

| Procedures |
| --- |
| MIS TLIF, MIS MIDLF |
| Radiographs unavailable |

| Supplemental fixation systems |
| --- |
| Globus Medical REVOLVE® Posterior Stabilization System |

**Table 6.4** Medtronic CD Horizon® Solera® Cortical Fixation Spinal System

| Design |
|---|
| **Set screw specifications**<br>Breakoff screws improve ease of insertion and final tightening<br>Standard threading eliminates difficulties of cross-threading |

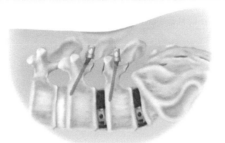

CD Horizon® Solera® cortical screw insertion

| Modular aspects and variations | | | |
|---|---|---|---|
| **Screw diameters**<br>4.5, 5, 6.5, 7.5 mm | **Screw lengths**<br>20–35 mm (5-mm increments),<br>40, 45 mm (6.5, 7.5 mm diameters) | **Rod type**<br>Prebent | **Rod lengths**<br>30–45 mm (5-mm increments),<br>50–80 mm (10-mm increments), 100 mm |

| Procedures |
|---|
| MIS TLIF, MIS MIDLF |
| Radiographs unavailable |

| Supplemental fixation systems |
|---|
| Medtronic CD Horizon® Solera® Posterior Stabilization System |

**Table 6.5** NuVasive MAS® PLIF Platform

| Design |
| --- |

**Set screw specifications**

Helical flange locking technology to reduce head splay and cross-threading

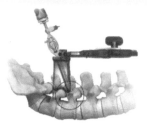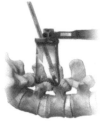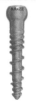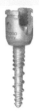

Shank insertion using Shank Driver and Screw Head Attachment with Head Inserter (far left and middle left), free-standing trizone shank (middle right), and free-standing polyaxial screw (far right)

| Modular aspects and variations | | | |
| --- | --- | --- | --- |
| **Screw diameters**<br>4.5, 5, 5.5, 6.5 mm | **Screw lengths**<br>25–40 mm (5-mm increments) | **Rod type**<br>Prebent<br>Straight | **Rod lengths**<br>20–100 mm (5-mm increments), 110, 120 mm |

| Procedures |
| --- |

MIS TLIF, MIS posterior decompression

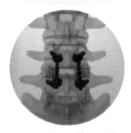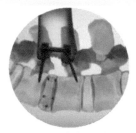

Anteroposterior and lateral illustrations of NuVasive MAS® PLIF Platform placement

| Supplemental fixation systems |
| --- |

NuVasive MaXcess® MAS® PLIF Access System, Precept® MAS® PLIF Fixation System, CoRoent® MAS® PLIF Interbody System

# References

[1] Santoni BG, Hynes RA, McGilvray KC, et al. Cortical bone trajectory for lumbar pedicle screws. Spine J. 2009; 9(5):366–373

[2] Sansur CA, Caffes NM, Ibrahimi DM, et al. Biomechanical fixation properties of cortical versus transpedicular screws in the osteoporotic lumbar spine: an in vitro human cadaveric model. J Neurosurg Spine. 2016; 25(4):467–476

[3] Chen YR, Deb S, Pham L, Singh H. Minimally invasive lumbar pedicle screw fixation using cortical bone trajectory: a prospective cohort study on postoperative pain outcomes. Cureus. 2016; 8(7):e714

[4] Calvert GC, Lawrence BD, Abtahi AM, Bachus KN, Brodke DS. Cortical screws used to rescue failed lumbar pedicle screw construct: a biomechanical analysis. J Neurosurg Spine. 2015; 22(2):166–172

[5] Lee GW, Son JH, Ahn MW, Kim HJ, Yeom JS. The comparison of pedicle screw and cortical screw in posterior lumbar interbody fusion: a prospective randomized noninferiority trial. Spine J. 2015; 15(7):1519–1526

[6] Baluch DA, Patel AA, Lullo B, et al. Effect of physiological loads on cortical and traditional pedicle screw fixation. Spine. 2014; 39(22):E1297–E1302

[7] Mizuno M, Kuraishi K, Umeda Y, Sano T, Tsuji M, Suzuki H. Midline lumbar fusion with cortical bone trajectory screw. Neurol Med Chir (Tokyo). 2014; 54(9):716–721

[8] Mobbs RJ. The "medio-latero-superior trajectory technique": an alternative cortical trajectory for pedicle fixation. Orthop Surg. 2013; 5(1):56–59

[9] Ueno M, Sakai R, Tanaka K, et al. Should we use cortical bone screws for cortical bone trajectory? J Neurosurg Spine. 2015; 22(4):416–421

[10] Inceoğlu S, Montgomery WH, Jr, St Clair S, McLain RF. Pedicle screw insertion angle and pullout strength: comparison of 2 proposed strategies. J Neurosurg Spine. 2011; 14(5):670–676

[11] Matsukawa K, Yato Y, Imabayashi H, Hosogane N, Asazuma T, Nemoto K. Biomechanical evaluation of the fixation strength of lumbar pedicle screws using cortical bone trajectory: a finite element study. J Neurosurg Spine. 2015; 23(4):471–478

[12] Matsukawa K, Yato Y, Kato T, Imabayashi H, Asazuma T, Nemoto K. In vivo analysis of insertional torque during pedicle screwing using cortical bone trajectory technique. Spine. 2014; 39(4):E240–E245

[13] Wray S, Mimran R, Vadapalli S, Shetye SS, McGilvray KC, Puttlitz CM. Pedicle screw placement in the lumbar spine: effect of trajectory and screw design on acute biomechanical purchase. J Neurosurg Spine. 2015; 22(5):503–510

[14] Patel SS, Cheng WK, Danisa OA. Early complications after instrumentation of the lumbar spine using cortical bone trajectory technique. J Clin Neurosci. 2016; 24:63–67

[15] Snyder LA, Martinez-Del-Campo E, Neal MT, et al. Lumbar spinal fixation with cortical bone trajectory pedicle screws in 79 patients with degenerative disease: perioperative outcomes and complications. World Neurosurg. 2016; 88:205–213

# 7 Facet Screw Systems

*Simon P. Lalehzarian, Benjamin Khechen, Brittany E. Haws, Kaitlyn L. Cardinal, Jordan A. Guntin, and Kern Singh*

## 7.1 Introduction

The posterior approach for facet screw fixation is described in Chapter 3 Posterior Retractor Systems. Facet screws were developed as an alternative to the standard pedicle screw fixation system.[1] By utilizing facet screws as an adjunct to minimally invasive fusion, the safety, feasibility, and overall morbidity associated with standard fixation were all theorized to substantially improve.[2] Surgical indications are presented in ▶ Table 7.1.

### 7.1.1 Facet Screw Components

Facet screws are similar in design to pedicle screws, with variations in body length to accommodate the different approach and point of fixation.[1] The "translaminar transfacet" and "transfacet pedicle" techniques were both developed to provide access to the facet joints for appropriate fixation (▶ Fig. 7.1).[3] Both techniques have exhibited successful restriction of facet motion; however, there are differences in the type of instrumentation and insertion angle utilized in each technique.[1] The translaminar transfacet technique utilizes longer screw lengths with the perceived benefit of increasing mechanical robustness.[2] This technique also utilizes a different angle of insertion in order to enter the contralateral lamina and end at the base of the ipsilateral transverse process, potentially increasing the strength of fixation.[3,4]

### 7.1.2 Outcomes

Facet screws have exhibited exceptional outcomes when utilized as a method of spinal fixation. These instruments have been demonstrated to induce stability in multiple spinal motion planes, including flexion, extension, and rotation.[5] Additionally, translaminar facet screws have been noted to increase the stiffness of spinal motion segments and the associated interbody device.[6,7,8] These characteristics are thought to reduce the risk of cage collapse and subsidence.[8] Furthermore, by stabilizing the facet joint, facet screws are able to minimize the uncoupling of the facet that occurs from interbody device distraction.[7,9] This consequently provides increased stability in extension and

**Table 7.1** Surgical indications for facet screws

| Indications |
| --- |
| • Anterior approach spinal fusion |
| • Posterior approach spinal fusion |
| • Cervical procedures |
| • Thoracolumbar procedures |
| • Degenerative disk disease |
| • Spondylolisthesis |
| • Spinal fracture/dislocation |
| • Spinal stenosis |

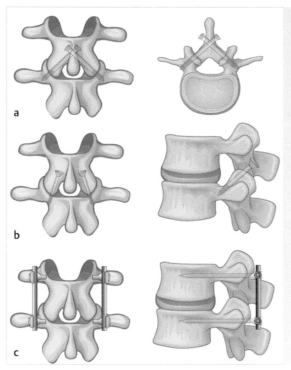

**Fig. 7.1** **(a)** Translaminar transfacet technique. **(b)** Transfacet pedicle technique. **(c)** Standard pedicle screw placement.

axial rotation, which is often weakened from interbody distraction.[9] Facet screws also exhibit advantages when compared to other types of spinal instrumentation. Previous studies have determined significant reduction in rates of neurologic injury and cerebrospinal fluid leaks with facet screw fixation in comparison to pedicle screw fixation.[10,11] Biomechanically, facet screws often appear to be equivalent to pedicle screws in providing mechanical fixation and stability.[5,8,12]

# 7.2 Facet Screw Systems

**Table 7.2** Alphatec Spine Illico® FS Facet Fixation System

| Design | |
| --- | --- |
| **Composition** | **Design feature** |
| Titanium alloy | Dual-lead thread design expedites screw implantation |

Facet screw insertion using a ratcheting axial handle attached to screw driver shaft (left) and upon insertion (right)

| Modular aspects and variations | |
| --- | --- |
| Facet screw specifications | |
| **Diameter** | **Lengths** |
| 4.5, 5 mm | 25–45 (5.0-mm increments), 35, 40 mm |

Cannulated screws available in fully (left) and partially threaded (right) designs

| Procedures |
| --- |

MIS TLIF, MIS posterior decompression

Radiographs unavailable

**Table 7.3** DePuy Synthes VIPER® F2 Facet Fixation System

| Design | |
| --- | --- |
| **Composition** Gold and silver | **Design feature** Dual-lead thread design expedites screw implantation |

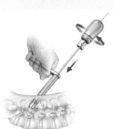 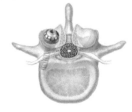 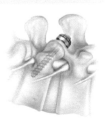

Screw and polyaxial ring insertion using cannulated self-retaining screwdriver (left) with final positioning (middle and right)

| Modular aspects and variations | | |
| --- | --- | --- |
| **Screw diameters** 5, 6 mm | **Screw lengths** 20–60 mm (5-mm increments) | **Washer diameter** 13, 16 mm |

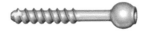  

Dual-lead cannulated threaded screw    Washer options for two piece polyaxial implant design

| Procedures |
| --- |

MIS TLIF, MIS posterior decompression

Radiographs unavailable

**Table 7.4** Globus Medical ZYFUSE® Facet Fixation System

| Design | |
|---|---|
| **Composition** | **Design features** |
| Titanium alloy | Dual-lead thread design expedites screw implantation |
| | Cannulated screws are hydroxyapatite coated to promote bone growth |

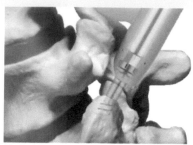

Globus Medical ZYFUSE® Facet Fixation System upon insertion

| Modular Aspects and Variations |
|---|

### Facet Screw Specifications

| Diameter | Lengths |
|---|---|
| 5, 6 mm | 30–60 mm (10-mm increments) |

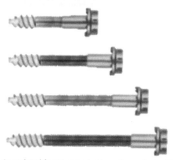

Cannulated facet screws (with washers attached)

| Procedures |
|---|

MIS TLIF, MIS posterior decompression

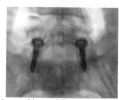 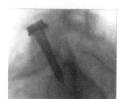

Anteroposterior and lateral fluoroscopic images of Globus Medical ZYFUSE® Facet Fixation System placement

**Table 7.5** Zimmer Biomet CONCERO™ Facet Screw System

| Design | |
|---|---|
| **Composition** | **Design feature** |
| Titanium alloy | Fixed lag length construct with dual-lead thread screw design |

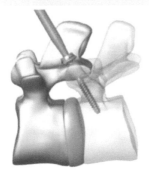 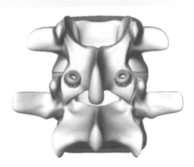

Screw insertion using facet screw driver (left) and final bilateral construct (right)

| Modular Aspects and Variations | | | |
|---|---|---|---|
| **Screw diameter** | **Screw lengths** | **Washer diameter** | **Washer height** |
| 4.5 mm | 25–45 mm (2.5-mm increments) | 11 mm | 4.75 mm |

| Procedures |
|---|
| MIS TLIF, MIS posterior decompression |
| No radiographs |

**Table 7.6** Zimmer Biomet LDR FacetBRIDGE™ Facet Fixation System

| Design | |
|---|---|
| **Composition** | **Design feature** |
| Titanium alloy | Comes preassembled as a screw and washer construct |

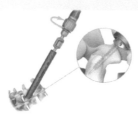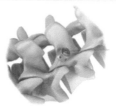

Screw insertion and washer placement using screwdriver and guidewire

| Modular aspects and variations | | | |
|---|---|---|---|
| **Screw diameters** | **Screw lengths** | **Washer diameter** | **Washer height** |
| 4.5, 5.5 mm | 15, 17.5, 20–55 mm (5-mm increments) | 12 mm | 5.5 mm |

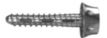

4.5-mm-diameter model          5.5-mm-diameter model

Fenestrated screw (with washer attached) eases insertion and permits the screw to self-fill

4.5-mm-diameter model          5.5-mm-diameter model

Fenestrated screw (with washer attached) eases insertion and permits the screw to self-fill

| Procedures |
|---|
| MIS TLIF, MIS posterior decompression |

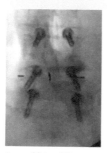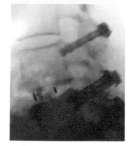

Anteroposterior and lateral fluoroscopic images of Zimmer Biomet FacetBRIDGE™ Facet Fixation System

# References

[1] Agarwala A, Bucklen B, Muzumdar A, Moldavsky M, Khalil S. Do facet screws provide the required stability in lumbar fixation? A biomechanical comparison of the Boucher technique and pedicular fixation in primary and circumferential fusions. Clin Biomech (Bristol, Avon). 2012; 27(1):64–70

[2] Ferrara LA, Secor JL, Jin BH, Wakefield A, Inceoglu S, Benzel EC. A biomechanical comparison of facet screw fixation and pedicle screw fixation: effects of short-term and long-term repetitive cycling. Spine. 2003; 28(12):1226–1234

[3] Best NM, Sasso RC. Efficacy of translaminar facet screw fixation in circumferential interbody fusions as compared to pedicle screw fixation. J Spinal Disord Tech. 2006; 19(2):98–103

[4] Lu J, Ebraheim NA, Yeasting RA. Translaminar facet screw placement: an anatomic study. Am J Orthop. 1998; 27(8):550–555

[5] Vanden Berghe L, Mehdian H, Lee AJ, Weatherley CR. Stability of the lumbar spine and method of instrumentation. Acta Orthop Belg. 1993; 59(2):175–180

[6] Heggeness MH, Esses SI. Translaminar facet joint screw fixation for lumbar and lumbosacral fusion. A clinical and biomechanical study. Spine. 1991; 16(6) Suppl:S266–S269

[7] Rathonyi GC, Oxland TR, Gerich U, Grassmann S, Nolte LP. The role of supplemental translaminar screws in anterior lumbar interbody fixation: a biomechanical study. Eur Spine J. 1998; 7(5):400–407

[8] Volkman T, Horton WC, Hutton WC. Transfacet screws with lumbar interbody reconstruction: biomechanical study of motion segment stiffness. J Spinal Disord. 1996; 9(5):425–432

[9] Lund T, Oxland TR, Jost B, et al. Interbody cage stabilisation in the lumbar spine: biomechanical evaluation of cage design, posterior instrumentation and bone density. J Bone Joint Surg Br. 1998; 80(2):351–359

[10] Grob D, Humke T. Translaminar screw fixation in the lumbar spine: technique, indications, results. Eur Spine J. 1998; 7(3):178–186

[11] Tuli J, Tuli S, Eichler ME, Woodard EJ. A comparison of long-term outcomes of translaminar facet screw fixation and pedicle screw fixation: a prospective study. J Neurosurg Spine. 2007; 7(3):287–292

[12] Deguchi M, Cheng BC, Sato K, Matsuyama Y, Zdeblick TA. Biomechanical evaluation of translaminar facet joint fixation. A comparative study of poly-L-lactide pins, screws, and pedicle fixation. Spine. 1998; 23(12):1307–1312, discussion 1313

# 8 Spinous Process Fixation Systems

*Jordan A. Guntin, Benjamin Khechen, Brittany E. Haws, Kaitlyn L. Cardinal, and Kern Singh*

## 8.1 Introduction

Spinous process fixation is another method utilized to provide spinal stability following interbody fusion. These devices are designed to provide additional stability through interspinous fusion.[1] Many interspinous fixation devices (IFDs) also provide interspinous process spacing, which can provide further decompression.[1] Additionally, the placement of this device only requires a single midline incision, which may make it a more expedient procedure compared to standard pedicle screw fixation. Surgical indications are presented in ▶ Table 8.1.

### 8.1.1 Interspinous Fixation Device Components

IFDs contain plates that clamp to the lateral aspects of adjacent spinous processes (▶ Fig. 8.1).[2] The clamps are often fixed to the spinous processes through the use of rivets or spiked plates. By securing segment motion posteriorly, an IFD can provide rigidity to the two adjacent vertebrae to which it is secured.[2] IFDs can be composed of a variety of materials, including polyetheretherketone (PEEK) and titanium.

**Table 8.1** Surgical indications for interspinous fixation devices

| Indications |
| --- |
| • Posterior approach spinal fusion |
| • Thoracic procedures |
| • Lumbosacral procedures |
| • Degenerative disk disease |
| • Spondylolisthesis |
| • Spinal fracture/dislocation |
| • Spinal tumor |

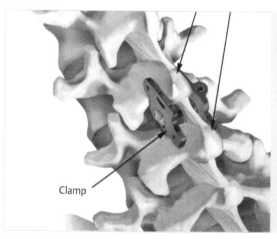

Clamp

**Fig. 8.1** Interspinous fixation device with clamps fixated on the spinous processes of two adjacent lumbar vertebrae. (Adapted from Aspen® MIS Fusion System Surgical Technique Guide, Zimmer Biomet, 2014.)

## 8.1.2 Outcomes

Spinous process fixation has exhibited promising outcomes with regard to its efficacy. Previous studies have demonstrated similar fusion rates when utilizing either supplemental spinous process fixation or pedicle screw fixation.[1,3,4] Additionally, IFDs have exhibited comparable rigidity to pedicle screws, especially in flexion–extension movements of the lumbar spine.[5,6] This is supplemented with evidence of reduced motion at adjacent segments, suggesting a reduced risk for adjacent segment disease when IFDs are utilized.[1] However, the literature is limited regarding high-quality comparative studies. Few studies have examined the complication profile of IFDs.[1] Furthermore, evidence regarding long-term outcomes and benefits of IFDs has not been addressed.[1] As such, the literature is inadequate to identify the true advantages of IFDs over other methods of fixation.

## 8.2 Spinous Process Fixation Systems

**Table 8.2** Alphatec Spine BridgePoint® Spinous Process Fixation System

| Design | | |
| --- | --- | --- |
| **Device type** | **Composition** | **Specifications** |
| Fixed | Titanium alloy | Angulating and telescoping plates enhance device fit and promote fusion |

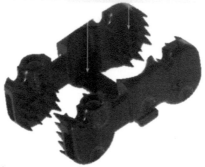

Alphatec BridgePoint® Spinous Process Fixation System

| Modular aspects and variations | | |
| --- | --- | --- |
| **Widths** | **Angulation** | **Compression/distraction** |
| Small: 35–40 mm | ±14° | Telescoping plates provide up to |
| Medium: 40–45 mm | | 5 mm adjustment |
| Large: 45–50 mm | | |

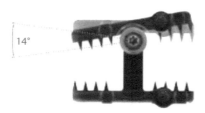

Telescoping plate angluation up to 14°

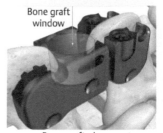

Bone graft placement

| Procedures |
| --- |
| MIS TLIF, MIS posterior decompression |
| Radiographs unavailable |
| **Supplemental fixation system** |
| Alphatec Spine Illico® Posterior Stabilization System |

**Table 8.3** Globus Medical SP-Fix™ Spinous Process Fixation Plate

| Design | | |
| --- | --- | --- |
| **Plate type** | **Composition** | **Specification** |
| Fixed | Titanium and PEEK | Zero-step locking mechanism expedites the implantation process |

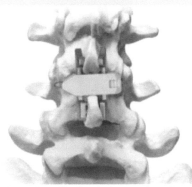

Interspinous fixation device upon insertion

| Modular aspects and variations | | | |
| --- | --- | --- | --- |
| **Rod sizes** | **Barrel heights** | **Plate lengths** | **Angulation** |
| 25, 30, 35 mm | 8–20 mm (2-mm increments) | 35–47 (3-mm increments), 50, 55 mm | ±15° |

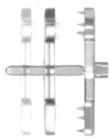

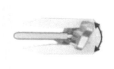 

Lateral and anterior views of plate and barrel assembly

Automatic locking as the implant is compressed

| Procedures |
| --- |
| MIS TLIF, MIS posterior decompression |
| Radiographs unavailable |

| Supplemental fixation system |
| --- |
| Globus Medical REVOLVE® Posterior Stabilization System |

**Table 8.4** NuVasive Affix® II Spinous Process Plate Device

| Design | | | |
|---|---|---|---|
| **Device type** | **Composition** | **Plate lengths** | **Specifications** |
| Fixed | Titanium alloy | 35–55 mm (10-mm increments) | One-step insertion and self-locking mechanism |

Affix II stand alone (left) and upon insertion (right)

| Procedures |
|---|
| MIS TLIF, MIS posterior decompression |
| Radiographs unavailable |

| Supplemental fixation system |
|---|
| NuVasive Precept® Posterior Stabilization System |

**Table 8.5** OsteoMed PrimaLOK™ SP Interspinous Fusion System

| Design | | |
|---|---|---|
| **Device type** | **Composition** | **Specifications** |
| Fixed | Titanium alloy | Polyaxial movement facilitates anterior placement |

Illustration of OsteoMed PrimaLOK™ SP polyaxial movement

| Modular aspects and variations | | | | | |
|---|---|---|---|---|---|
| **Height (A)** | **Width (B)** | **Grip distance (C)** | **Length (D)** | **Width (E)** | **Central post length** |
| 8–12 mm | 5.5–13.5 mm | 39 mm | 17 mm | | |
| (2-mm | 5.5–13.5 mm | 28 mm | 45 mm | 17 mm | 25 and 30 mm |
| increments) | | 34 mm | | | 25 and 30 mm |
| 15–18 mm | | | | | |
| (3-mm | | | | | |
| increments) | | | | | |

Anterior and lateral views of PrimaLOK SP Interspinous Fusion System

| Procedures |
|---|
| MIS TLIF, decompression |
| Radiographs unavailable |

| Supplemental fixation system |
|---|
| OsteoMed MIS Posterior Stabilization System |

**Table 8.6** Paradigm Spine Coflex® Interlaminar Technology

| Design | | |
| --- | --- | --- |
| **Device type** | **Composition** | **Specifications** |
| Fixed | Titanium alloy | In situ compressible in extension, which allows for flexion upon insertion |

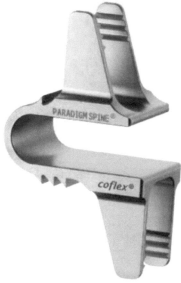

Paradigm Spine Coflex® Interlaminar device shown as free-standing construct

| Modular aspects and variations | |
| --- | --- |
| **Available sizes** | **Distal arm length** |
| 8–16 mm (2-mm increments) | 5–13 mm (2-mm increments) |

**Table 8.6** (*Continued*) Paradigm Spine Coflex® Interlaminar Technology

### Procedures

MIS TLIF, MIS posterior decompression

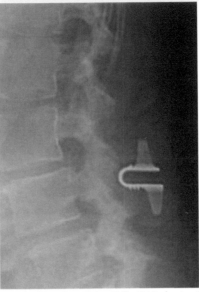

Lateral radiograph of Paradigm Spine Coflex® Interlaminar Technology ·

### Supplemental fixation system

Paradigm Spine MIS Posterior Stabilization System

**Table 8.7** RTI Surgical BacFuse® Spinous Process Fusion Plate System

| Design | | |
| --- | --- | --- |
| **Device type** | **Composition** | **Specifications** |
| Fixed | Titanium alloy | Torque-controlled locking mechanism confirms fixation |

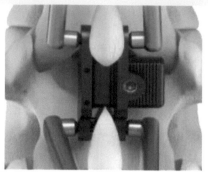

RTI Surgical BacFuse® illustrated while under compression

| Modular aspects and variations | | | | |
| --- | --- | --- | --- | --- |
| **Caudal-cranial length** | **Maximum width** | **Barrel height** | **A/P length** | **Angulation** |
| 35–37 mm (0.5-mm increments) | 12.5 mm | 8–16 mm (2-mm increments) | 16 mm | ±10° |

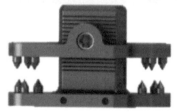 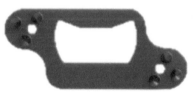

RTI Surgical BacFuse® fully constructed (left) and plate (right)

| Procedures |
| --- |
| MIS TLIF, MIS posterior decompression |
| Radiographs unavailable |

| Supplemental fixation system |
| --- |
| RTI Surgical MIS Posterior Stabilization System |

**Table 8.8** SeaSpine Spinous Process Fixation System

| Design | | | |
| --- | --- | --- | --- |
| **Device type** | **Composition** | **Available sizes** | **Angulation** |
| Fixed | Titanium alloy | 6–16 mm (2-mm increments) | ±10° |

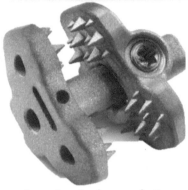

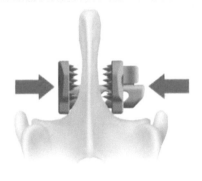

Aggressive spikes for secure fixation      Ratchet mechanism maintains compression

| Procedures |
| --- |
| MIS TLIF, MIS posterior decompression |

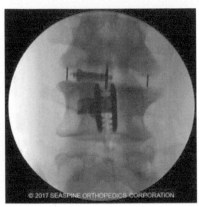

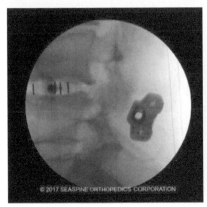

Anteroposterior and lateral fluoroscopic images of SeaSpine Spinous Process Fixation System

| Supplemental fixation system |
| --- |
| SeaSpine Spinous Process MIS Posterior Stabilization System |

**Table 8.9** Stryker UniVise® Spinous Process Fixation Plate System

| Design | | | |
| --- | --- | --- | --- |
| **Device type** | **Composition** | **Specifications** | **Available sizes** |
| Fixed | Titanium alloy | Midline approach with centralized locking mechanism | 35 and 40 mm |

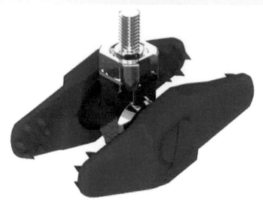

Illustration of Stryker UniVise® Spinous Process Fixation Plate System one-piece design with a radial spike pattern

| Procedures |
| --- |
| MIS TLIF, MIS posterior decompression |
| Radiographs unavailable |
| **Supplemental fixation system** |
| Stryker UniVise® MIS Posterior Stabilization System |

**Table 8.10** Zimmer Biomet ALPINE XC™ Adjustable Fusion System

| Design | | |
| --- | --- | --- |
| **Device type** | **Composition** | **Specifications** |
| Expandable | Titanium | Adjustability allows in situ distraction and compression |

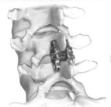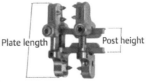

Zimmer Biomet ALPINE XC™ upon insertion and free standing

| Modular aspects and variations | | |
| --- | --- | --- |
| **Post length** | **Post height range** | **Ventral graft containment** |
| Medium (21 mm) | 6–18 mm | Medium: 6–12 mm |
| Wide (24 mm) | 10–18 mm | Wide: 10–18 mm |

| Procedures |
| --- |
| MIS TLIF, MIS posterior decompression |

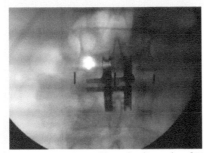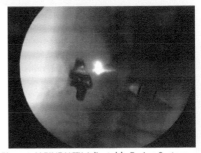

Anteroposterior and lateral radiographs of Zimmer Biomet ALPINE XC™ Adjustable Fusion System

| Supplemental fixation system |
| --- |
| Zimmer Biomet MIS Posterior Stabilization System |

**Table 8.11** Zimmer Biomet ASPEN® MIS Fusion System

| Design | | |
|---|---|---|
| **Device type** | **Composition** | **Specifications** |
| Fixed | Titanium and cobalt | Models designed for specific spinal levels |

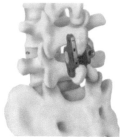
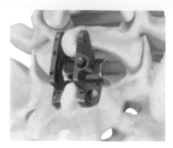

ASPEN® medium implant upon insertion    ASPEN® flared 5–1 implant upon insertion at L5–S1

| Modular aspects and variations | | | | |
|---|---|---|---|---|
| **Type** | **Width options** | **Barrel length** | **Angulation** | **Offset** |
| Standard | 8–18 mm (2-mm increments) | 21 mm | 10° | – |
| Medium | 6–14 mm (2-mm increments) | 18 mm | 10° | – |
| Flared 5–1 (special order) | 8–18 mm (2-mm increments) | – | 10° | 45° |

Illustration of the standard (left), medium (middle), and flared 5–1 (right) implant

| Procedures |
|---|
| MIS TLIF, MIS posterior decompression |

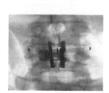

Anteroposterior and lateral fluoroscopic images of Zimmer Biomet ASPEN® MIS Fusion System

| Supplemental fixation system |
|---|
| Zimmer Biomet MIS Posterior Stabilization System |

# References

[1] Lopez AJ, Scheer JK, Dahdaleh NS, et al. Lumbar spinous process fixation and fusion: a systematic review and critical analysis of an emerging spinal technology. Clin Spine Surg. 2017; 30(9):E1279–E1288

[2] Gazzeri R, Galarza M, Alfieri A. Controversies about interspinous process devices in the treatment of degenerative lumbar spine diseases: past, present, and future. BioMed Res Int. 2014; 2014:975052

[3] Vokshoor A, Khurana S, Wilson D, Filsinger P. Clinical and radiographic outcomes after spinous process fixation and posterior fusion in an elderly cohort. Surg Technol Int. 2014; 25:271–276

[4] Kim HJ, Bak KH, Chun HJ, Oh SJ, Kang TH, Yang MS. Posterior interspinous fusion device for one-level fusion in degenerative lumbar spine disease: comparison with pedicle screw fixation—preliminary report of at least one year follow up. J Korean Neurosurg Soc. 2012; 52(4):359–364

[5] Gonzalez-Blohm SA, Doulgeris JJ, Aghayev K, Lee WE, III, Volkov A, Vrionis FD. Biomechanical analysis of an interspinous fusion device as a stand-alone and as supplemental fixation to posterior expandable interbody cages in the lumbar spine. J Neurosurg Spine. 2014; 20(2):209–219

[6] Techy F, Mageswaran P, Colbrunn RW, Bonner TF, McLain RF. Properties of an interspinous fixation device (ISD) in lumbar fusion constructs: a biomechanical study. Spine J. 2013; 13(5):572–579

**Part II**

**Lateral Approach**

9  Introduction to MIS
   Lateral Approach          *120*

10 Lateral Retractor
   Systems                   *126*

11 Lateral Interbody
   Cages                     *133*

12 Lateral Fixation
   Systems                   *145*

13 Vertebral Body Repla-
   cement Devices            *156*

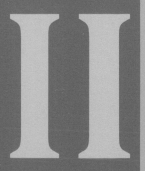

# 9 Introduction to MIS Lateral Approach

*Sravisht Iyer, Benjamin Khechen, Brittany E. Haws, Jordan A. Guntin, Kaitlyn L. Cardinal, and Kern Singh*

## 9.1 Introduction

The lateral minimally invasive surgery (MIS) approach was developed with the goal of reduced morbidity when compared to the anterior and posterior approaches to lumbar interbody fusion.[1,2] Compared to the posterior approach, lateral access provides direct visualization of the disk space without requiring direct entry into the spinal canal or retraction of neural elements.[3,4] Furthermore, the MIS lateral approach allows for placement of interbody devices with larger footprints.[1,5]

## 9.2 Surgical Anatomy

Superficial anatomical landmarks for orientation include the 12th rib, pubic symphysis, and the lateral border of the rectus abdominis. Musculature encountered in this approach, from superficial to deep, includes the external oblique, internal oblique, transversus abdominis, and psoas. Blunt dissection and traversal of the external oblique, internal oblique, and transversus abdominis muscles are not typically associated with significant morbidity, as they are segmentally innervated and denervation is unlikely to occur.

The most significant anatomic concern is transient or permanent neural injury during traversal and retraction of the psoas musculature.[6,7] Branches of the lumbar plexus are located within the posterior aspect of the psoas, and consequently these structures can be injured by retraction if they are in close proximity to the surgical corridor (▶ Fig. 9.1). This risk is increased at more caudal levels, with the plexus lying more anteriorly and thus closer to the surgical corridor at the L4–L5 level.[8,9] As the risk for neurologic injury is concerning, the use of neuromonitoring during traversal and retraction of the psoas is necessary to identify a safe working zone. Furthermore, the risk of injury to the contralateral retroperitoneal vasculature is also higher at more caudal levels such as L4–L5.[8] At these levels, the vasculature is located more posteriorly with greater overlap of the anterior disk space. With greater disk space overlap, the vasculature has a higher likelihood of injury during contralateral annulotomy.

## 9.3 Surgical Technique

### 9.3.1 Positioning

Proper positioning is essential during the lateral approach so as to ensure that the surgical plane is perpendicular to the disk space.[10] Patients are placed on a radiolucent table in the lateral decubitus position with the operative site positioned over the break in the bed to ensure maximal flexion at the surgical level (▶ Fig. 9.2). In some cases, the table can be retroflexed to increase the distance between the iliac crest and ribs, while the hips can also be moderately flexed to promote psoas muscle relaxation.[1,11] The pelvis and thorax are secured with tape and the arms are well padded. Use of an axillary roll also aids in preventing the incidence of brachial plexopathies. The C-arm and surgical monitor should be placed on the side opposite to the surgeon for optimal viewing.

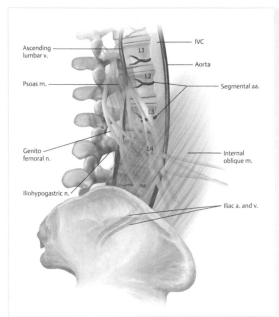

**Fig. 9.1** Illustration depicting the positional relationship of lumbar plexus branches and surrounding musculature. (Adapted from An H, Singh K, eds. Synopsis of Spine Surgery. 3rd ed. New York, NY: Thieme; 2016.)

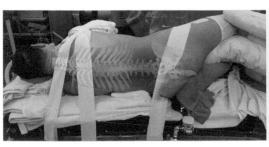

**Fig. 9.2** Lateral decubitus positioning for MIS lateral approach. (Adapted from Singh K, ed. Spine Essentials Handbook: A Bulleted Review of Anatomy, Evaluation, Imaging, Tests, and Procedures. New York, NY: Thieme; 2019.)

Electromyographic (EMG) neuromonitoring is typically used in the lateral approach as branches of the lumbar plexus can be encountered upon traversal of the psoas muscle.[10]

## 9.3.2 Approach

The initial descriptions of the lateral lumbar interbody fusion (LLIF) utilized a two-incision approach with a more posterior approach to confirm retroperitoneal positioning prior to deep dissection.[1] However, single-incision approaches are now commonly utilized. The lateral incision is placed using fluoroscopic imaging. The abdominal musculature including the external oblique, internal oblique, and transversalis fascia should be bluntly dissected until the retroperitoneum is entered (▶ Fig. 9.3). Once the surgeon has confirmed he or she is in the retroperitoneal space, finger dissection is carried to the lateral surface of the psoas. Serial dilators are then introduced to the disk space through the psoas muscle using fluoroscopy to confirm appropriate placement. Free-running EMG monitoring is used to ensure that the lumbar plexus is not inadvertently

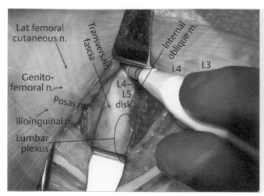

**Fig. 9.3** Intraoperative photograph demonstrating dissection of the internal oblique muscle and identification of the transversalis fascia and underlying retroperitoneal space. (Adapted from Singh K, Vaccaro A, eds. Pocket Atlas of Spine Surgery. 2nd ed. New York, NY: Thieme; 2018.)

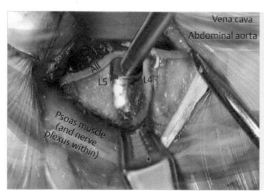

**Fig. 9.4** Intraoperative photograph demonstrating endplate preparation. (Adapted from Singh K, Vaccaro A, eds. Pocket Atlas of Spine Surgery. 2nd ed. New York, NY: Thieme; 2018.)

injured.[12,13] The dilators are then docked to the disk space and secured using a table-mounted retraction system. A fiberoptic light system is then attached to the retractor system to assist with visualization. A self-retaining retractor is then placed, with confirmation of correct localization via anteroposterior (AP) and lateral fluoroscopic views.

### 9.3.3 Disk Space Preparation

Bipolar cautery is used to expose the disk space and remove any residual tissue blocking visualization. An annulotomy is then performed, with removal of disk space material using curets, pituitaries, and rasps.[14] The annulotomy should be extended to the contralateral side to ensure adequate exposure and correction of coronal plane deformities. The end plates are prepared by removal of cartilaginous tissue using a combination of straight and curved curets (▶ Fig. 9.4).

### 9.3.4 Interbody Cage Placement

Next, a series of trial sizers are placed under fluoroscopic guidance. Once appropriate sizing has been achieved, the final interbody implant supplemented with an osteobiologic/graft enhancer such as recombinant human bone morphogenetic protein-2 (rhBMP-2) is impacted into the disk space under fluoroscopic guidance. The cage should span the entire width of the vertebral body, thus resting on the ring apophysis and reducing the incidence of subsidence. Final confirmation of cage placement is confirmed via AP and lateral fluoroscopy (▶ Fig. 9.5).

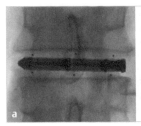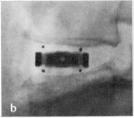

Fig. 9.5 (a) Anteroposterior and (b) lateral fluoroscopic images of lateral interbody cage placement. (Reproduced with permission of © Globus Medical Caliber – L Surgical Guide.)

### 9.3.5 Supplemental Fixation

When deemed clinically necessary, a variety of supplemental fixation techniques can be employed. Lateral plating can be performed through the initial incision, while placement of pedicle screws can be done with or without repositioning.[2,15]

### 9.3.6 Closure

The wound is copiously irrigated after confirmation of interbody cage placement. The incision is closed in layers, with subsequent application of dermabond and a sterile dressing. Long-acting local anesthetics can be injected intramuscularly to reduce postoperative pain.

## 9.4 Complications

The most important potential complication of LLIF is neurologic injury. Lykissas et al reported that a significant number of patients had postoperative thigh pain and sensory and motor deficits following LLIF.[16] In a series of 451 patients and 919 levels, the authors reported thigh pain in 39%, sensory deficit in 38%, and weakness in 24% of these patients in the immediate postoperative period. These were typically transient neuropraxias and these rates deduced to sensory deficit (usually anterior thigh) in 9.6% and weakness in 3.2% of patients by 18 months. Generally speaking, the reported rates of sensory deficits after LLIF range from 2.2 to 19.7% and the rates of motor deficits range from 0.7 to 8.9%.[5,11,12,13,14] Motor deficits may involve quadriceps weakness due to injury to the femoral nerve or hip flexor weakness due to dissection.

Lykissas et al demonstrated that the rates of early complications were associated with surgery at the L4–L5 level.[16] This is not entirely surprising given the anatomy of the lumbar plexus in the psoas muscle. Regev et al performed a MRI study showing that the lumbar plexus nerve roots moved anterior in the lower lumbar spine. The authors identified a "safe zone" for LLIF between the blood vessels anteriorly and the nerve roots posteriorly. In their analysis, this safe zone decreased from roughly 40 to 45% of the vertebral AP diameter in the upper lumbar spine (L1–L2 to L3–L4) to only 13% at L4–L5.[18] These findings have since been corroborated in cadaveric dissections as well.[17]

As with all procedures, the LLIF is associated with a surgical learning curve and there is evidence to suggest that the rate of neurologic complications decreases as surgeons gain more experience.[11] The impact of neurologic monitoring on avoiding these complications is unknown.

Vascular injury with LLIF is a rare but important complication to recognize as the consequences can be life-threatening.

## 9.5 Outcomes

LLIF offers an MIS approach to treat a variety of degenerative spine conditions such as spinal stenosis, degenerative spondylolisthesis, and degenerative scoliosis. Phillips et al were among the first to report on the utility of LLIF in patients with degenerative scoliosis. In a series of 107 patients, the authors reported improvement in pain, disability, and general health measures at 2-year follow up.[18] The authors also reported small corrections in the coronal and sagittal alignment. Similarly, in a series of 71 patients, Anand et al reported improvements in the sagittal balance and Cobb angle in patients with degenerative scoliosis with LLIF.[19] Both these studies, however, treated deformities that were small in magnitude (mean coronal Cobb 21–25 degrees). In patients with other degenerative conditions such as spinal stenosis and degenerative spondylolisthesis, LLIF has been associated with 30 to 70% improvement in the Visual Analog Scale (VAS) and Oswestry Disability Index (ODI) scores on average.[2,3,5,6 7]

LLIF has also been associated with significant improvements in the anterior and posterior disk height and cross-sectional foraminal area.[8,9] Radiographic fusion is readily achieved after LLIF, with reported rates between 88 and 100%.[17,20,21,22] Isaacs et al, in a study of 29 patients undergoing LLIF and 26 patients undergoing transforaminal lumbar interbody fusion (TLIF), analyzed and compared radiographic outcomes in both cohorts.[21] The LLIF group demonstrated significant improvements in overall disk height, along with significant improvements in ipsilateral and contralateral foraminal height postoperatively. However, increases in the central canal area were significantly lower in the LLIF group compared to the TLIF group (4.1 vs. 43.1 mm), possibly indicating the superiority of MIS TLIF in indirect neural decompression. In a systematic review of 21 investigations, Phan et al demonstrated significant improvements in coronal alignment after LLIF procedures.[23] From preoperative to final postoperative time points, the average coronal segmental cobb angle decreased from 3.6 to 1.1 degrees, while the average coronal regional cobb angle decreased from 19.1 to 10.0 degrees. However, only limited improvement was seen in sagittal alignment, as measured by preoperative and postoperative lumbar lordosis. Additional studies are required to fully elucidate the trends in radiographic improvement after interbody procedures via the MIS lateral approach.

Clinical outcomes as pertaining to spine-specific patient-reported measures have been extensively utilized to demonstrate the efficacy of the MIS lateral approach.[21,22,23,24,25,26] Ahmadian et al, in a multicenter study of 59 patients undergoing stand-alone LLIF, demonstrated significant improvements in pain and disability postoperatively.[22] At an average follow-up of 14.6 months, the VAS pain scores improved by 45.3%, while the ODI scores improved by 38.6%. Furthermore, fusion rate within this cohort was 93%. Sembrano et al, in a study of 29 patients undergoing LLIF with supplemental fixation, demonstrated similarly significant improvements in patient-reported outcomes.[24] At 24 months postoperatively, average improvements in the VAS pain, ODI, and 36-Item Short Form Survey (SF-36) scores were 73, 53, and 64%, respectively.

## References

[1] Pawar A, Hughes A, Girardi F, Sama A, Lebl D, Cammisa F. Lateral lumbar interbody fusion. Asian Spine J. 2015; 9(6):978–983

[2] Lehmen JA, Gerber EJ. MIS lateral spine surgery: a systematic literature review of complications, outcomes, and economics. Eur Spine J. 2015; 24 Suppl 3:287–313

[3] Rihn JA, Patel R, Makda J, et al. Complications associated with single-level transforaminal lumbar interbody fusion. Spine J. 2009; 9(8):623–629

[4] Potter BK, Freedman BA, Verwiebe EG, Hall JM, Polly DW, Jr, Kuklo TR. Transforaminal lumbar interbody fusion: clinical and radiographic results and complications in 100 consecutive patients. J Spinal Disord Tech. 2005; 18(4):337–346

[5] Kwon B, Kim DH. Lateral lumbar interbody fusion: indications, outcomes, and complications. J Am Acad Orthop Surg. 2016; 24(2):96–105

[6] Yuan PS, Rowshan K, Verma RB, Miller LE, Block JE. Minimally invasive lateral lumbar interbody fusion with direct psoas visualization. J Orthop Surg Res. 2014; 9:20

[7] Guérin P, Obeid I, Bourghli A, et al. The lumbosacral plexus: anatomic considerations for minimally invasive retroperitoneal transpsoas approach. Surg Radiol Anat. 2012; 34(2):151–157

[8] Regev GJ, Chen L, Dhawan M, Lee YP, Garfin SR, Kim CW. Morphometric analysis of the ventral nerve roots and retroperitoneal vessels with respect to the minimally invasive lateral approach in normal and deformed spines. Spine. 2009; 34(12):1330–1335

[9] Kepler CK, Bogner EA, Herzog RJ, Huang RC. Anatomy of the psoas muscle and lumbar plexus with respect to the surgical approach for lateral transpsoas interbody fusion. Eur Spine J. 2011; 20(4):550–556

[10] Winder MJ, Gambhir S. Comparison of ALIF vs. XLIF for L4/5 interbody fusion: pros, cons, and literature review. J Spine Surg. 2016; 2(1):2–8

[11] Yson SC, Sembrano JN, Santos ER, Luna JT, Polly DW, Jr. Does prone repositioning before posterior fixation produce greater lordosis in lateral lumbar interbody fusion (LLIF)? J Spinal Disord Tech. 2014; 27(7):364–369

[12] Banagan K, Gelb D, Poelstra K, Ludwig S. Anatomic mapping of lumbar nerve roots during a direct lateral transpsoas approach to the spine: a cadaveric study. Spine. 2011; 36(11):E687–E691

[13] Uribe JS, Vale FL, Dakwar E. Electromyographic monitoring and its anatomical implications in minimally invasive spine surgery. Spine. 2010; 35(26) Suppl:S368–S374

[14] Baaj AA. Handbook of Spine Surgery. New York, NY: Thieme; 2012

[15] Lehman A, Rodgers WB. Minimally disruptive lateral transpsoas approach for thoracolumbar anterior interbody fusion. In: Phillips FM, Lieberman IH, Polly DW Jr., Wang MY, eds. Minimally Invasive Spine Surgery: Surgical Techniques and Disease Management. New York, NY: Springer; 2014:167–190

[16] Lykissas MG, Aichmair A, Hughes AP, Sama AA, Lebl DR, Taher F, Du JY, Cammisa FP, Girardi FP. Nerve injury after lateral lumbar interbody fusion: a review of 919 treated levels with identification of risk factors. Spine J. 2014 May 1;14(5):749–758

[17] Waddell B, Briski D, Qadir R, et al. Lateral lumbar interbody fusion for the correction of spondylolisthesis and adult degenerative scoliosis in high-risk patients: early radiographic results and complications. Ochsner J. 2014; 14(1):23–31

[18] Phillips FM, Isaacs RE, Rodgers WB, Khajavi K, Tohmeh AG, Deviren V, Peterson MD, Hyde J, Kurd M. Adult degenerative scoliosis treated with XLIF: clinical and radiographical results of a prospective multicenter study with 24-month follow-up. Spine (Phila Pa 1976). 2013 Oct 1;38(21):1853–1861

[19] Anand N, Baron EM, Khandehroo B, Kahwaty S. Long-term 2- to 5-year clinical and functional outcomes of minimally invasive surgery for adult scoliosis. Spine (Phila Pa 1976). 2013 Aug 15;38(18):1566–1575

[20] Kotwal S, Kawaguchi S, Lebl D, et al. minimally invasive lateral lumbar interbody fusion: clinical and radiographic outcome at a minimum 2-year follow-up. J Spinal Disord Tech. 2015; 28(4):119–125

[21] Isaacs RE, Sembrano JN, Tohmeh AG, SOLAS Degenerative Study Group. Two-year comparative outcomes of MIS lateral and MIS transforaminal interbody fusion in the treatment of degenerative spondylolisthesis: part II: radiographic findings. Spine. 2016; 41 Suppl 8:S133–S144

[22] Ahmadian A, Bach K, Bolinger B, et al. Stand-alone minimally invasive lateral lumbar interbody fusion: multicenter clinical outcomes. J Clin Neurosci. 2015; 22(4):740–746

[23] Phan K, Rao PJ, Scherman DB, Dandie G, Mobbs RJ. Lateral lumbar interbody fusion for sagittal balance correction and spinal deformity. J Clin Neurosci. 2015; 22(11):1714–1721

[24] Sembrano JN, Tohmeh A, Isaacs R, SOLAS Degenerative Study Group. Two-year comparative outcomes of MIS lateral and MIS transforaminal interbody fusion in the treatment of degenerative spondylolisthesis: part I: clinical findings. Spine. 2016; 41 Suppl 8:S123–S132

[25] Ozgur BM, Agarwal V, Nail E, Pimenta L. Two-year clinical and radiographic success of minimally invasive lateral transpsoas approach for the treatment of degenerative lumbar conditions. SAS J. 2010; 4(2):41–46

[26] Ahmadian A, Verma S, Mundis GM, Jr, Oskouian RJ, Jr, Smith DA, Uribe JS. Minimally invasive lateral retroperitoneal transpsoas interbody fusion for L4–5 spondylolisthesis: clinical outcomes. J Neurosurg Spine. 2013; 19(3):314–320

# 10 Lateral Retractor Systems

*Mohammed Abbas, Benjamin Khechen, Brittany E. Haws, Jordan A. Guntin, Kaitlyn L. Cardinal, and Kern Singh*

## 10.1 Introduction

Of the various minimally invasive surgery (MIS) approaches, the lateral transpsoas approach has been extensively studied in regard to complications related to surgical exposure. During this approach, retraction systems traverse the psoas muscle, placing the psoas muscle and lumbar plexus at considerable risk of injury. Symptoms are typically transient and include thigh pain, groin pain, paresthesias, numbness, hip flexor weakness, and psoas spasm.[1,2,3,4,5,6,7,8,9] Avoidance of complications can be mediated by proper placement of tubular dilators and retraction systems. Additionally, the use of real-time neuromonitoring has reduced the incidence of neurologic injury via detection of nearby neural structures and subsequent adjustment of the approach by the surgeon.[10,11]

## 10.2 Lateral Retractor Systems

**Table 10.1** DePuy Synthes INSIGHT® Lateral Access System

| Retractor design | | |
|---|---|---|
| **Retractor system**<br>Expandable | **Retractor apparatus**<br>Dual tubular blades | **Design feature**<br>Bifurcated direct light source |
| | | |
| Winglets reduce anterior tissue creep | | Disk anchor blade improves stability |
| **Specifications** | | |
| **Blade winglets**<br>Length extension up to 10 mm<br>Width extension up to 7 mm | **Tubular blades**<br>Lengths: 80–180 mm (10-mm increments)<br>Toeing: up to 20° angulation | **Posterior disk anchor blade**<br>Lengths: 80–160 mm (10-mm increments) |
| **Procedure** | | |
| MIS LLIF, MIS decompression<br>Radiographs unavailable | | |
| **Compatible device** | | |
| DePuy Synthes COUGAR® LS Lateral Cage System | | |

**Table 10.2** Globus Medical MARS™ 3V Minimal Access Retractor System

| Design | | |
| --- | --- | --- |
| **Retractor system** | **Retractor apparatus** | **Design feature** |
| Expandable | Tubular blade | 4th blade attachment, widening and lengthening shims to reduce muscle creep |

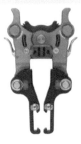 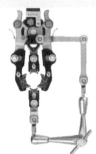

MARS™ 3V Expandable Retractor available in 2-blade (left) and 3-blade (right) models, with an available 4th blade attachment (right)

| Specifications | | |
| --- | --- | --- |
| **Posterior and cephalad–caudal blade lengths** 40–170 mm (10-mm increments) | **Port composition** Polyetheretherketone (PEEK) | **Angulation** Up to 20° independent blade angulation |

| Procedures |
| --- |
| MIS LLIF, MIS decompression |
| Radiographs unavailable |

| Compatible devices |
| --- |
| Globus Medical Lateral Fusion Systems |

**Table 10.3** K2 M RAVINE® Lateral Access System

| Retractor design | | |
| --- | --- | --- |
| **Retractor system** Expandable | **Retractor apparatus** Dual flat blade platform | **Design feature** Polyetheretherketone (PEEK) port composition |

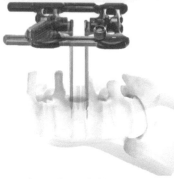

Enters the psoas in line with muscle fibers and fixates directly to the spine

| Specifications | | |
| --- | --- | --- |
| **Blade diameters** Flat blades: 24 mm Anteroposterior (AP) blades: 13 mm | **Flat blades** Lengths: 80–160 mm (10-mm increments) | **AP blades** Lengths: 80–160 mm (10-mm increments) |

| Procedure |
| --- |
| MIS LLIF, MIS decompression |

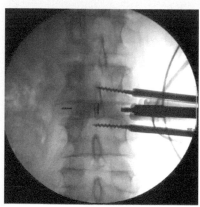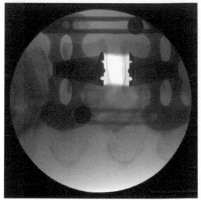

AP and lateral fluoroscopic images of K2M RAVINE® Lateral Access System

| Compatible devices |
| --- |
| K2 M ALEUTIAN® Lateral Interbody System |

**Table 10.4** NuVasive MaXcess® 4 Access System

| Retractor design | | |
|---|---|---|
| **Retractor system**<br>Expandable | **Retractor apparatus**<br>Tubular blade | **Design feature**<br>Locking intradiskal shim<br>improves retractor stability |

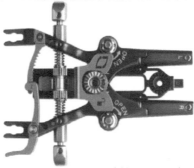

NuVasive MaXcess® 4 expandable retractor shown

| Specifications | |
|---|---|
| **Tubular blade lengths**<br>50–160 mm (10-mm increments) | **Dilator diameters**<br>6, 9, and 12 mm |

| Procedures |
|---|
| MIS LLIF, MIS decompression |

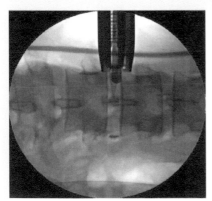 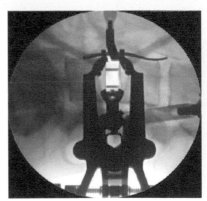

Anteroposterior and lateral fluoroscopic images of NuVasive MaXcess® Access System

| Compatible devices |
|---|
| NuVasive CoRoent® XL Platform, StruXureTM XLIF decade |

**Table 10.5** Zimmer Biomet AccuVision® Minimally Invasive Spinal Exposure System

| Retractor design | | |
| --- | --- | --- |
| **Retractor system**<br>Expandable | **Retractor apparatus**<br>Flat blade | **Design feature**<br>Supplemental retractor module provides additional mediolateral exposure |

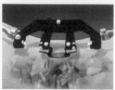 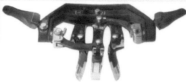 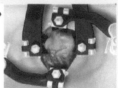

AccuVision® Minimally Invasive Spinal Exposure System retractor illustrated free-standing and upon insertion

| Specifications | | |
| --- | --- | --- |
| **Tubular blade widths and lengths**<br>18 mm × 40–110 mm (10-mm increments)<br>25 mm × 40–110 mm (10-mm increments) | **Flat blade lengths**<br>40–110 mm (10-mm increments) | **Dilator diameters**<br>7, 12, 18, 22, 25 mm |

| Procedures |
| --- |
| MIS LLIF, MIS decompression |
| Radiographs unavailable |

| Compatible devices |
| --- |
| Zimmer Biomet Lateral Fixation Systems |

**Table 10.6** Zimmer Biomet Timberline® Lateral Fusion System

| Retractor design | | |
| --- | --- | --- |
| **Retractor system** | **Retractor apparatus** | **Design feature** |
| Expandable | Tubular blade | Integrated posterior shim reduces retractor migration |

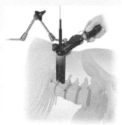

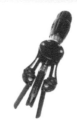

| | |
| --- | --- |
| Rotation of cephalad–caudal handle results in 17 mm of retraction | Individual blade movement improves access |

| Specifications | |
| --- | --- |
| **Posterior blade lengths** | **Cephalad–caudal blade lengths** |
| 50–180 mm (10-mm increments) | 50–180 mm (10-mm increments) |
| Toeing: Up to 20° angulation | Up to 17 mm of retraction |

| Procedures |
| --- |
| MIS LLIF, MIS decompression |

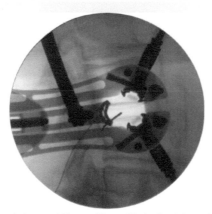

Lateral fluoroscopic image of Zimmer Biomet Timberline® Lateral Fusion System

| Compatible devices |
| --- |
| Zimmer Biomet Lateral Fusion Systems |

# References

[1] Youssef JA, McAfee PC, Patty CA, et al. Minimally invasive surgery: lateral approach interbody fusion: results and review. Spine. 2010; 35(26) Suppl:S302–S311

[2] Isaacs RE, Hyde J, Goodrich JA, Rodgers WB, Phillips FM. A prospective, nonrandomized, multicenter evaluation of extreme lateral interbody fusion for the treatment of adult degenerative scoliosis: perioperative outcomes and complications. Spine. 2010; 35(26) Suppl:S322–S330

[3] Cummock MD, Vanni S, Levi AD, Yu Y, Wang MY. An analysis of postoperative thigh symptoms after minimally invasive transpsoas lumbar interbody fusion. J Neurosurg Spine. 2011; 15(1):11–18

[4] Moller DJ, Slimack NP, Acosta FL, Jr, Koski TR, Fessler RG, Liu JC. Minimally invasive lateral lumbar interbody fusion and transpsoas approach-related morbidity. Neurosurg Focus. 2011; 31(4):E4

[5] Bergey DL, Villavicencio AT, Goldstein T, Regan JJ. Endoscopic lateral transpsoas approach to the lumbar spine. Spine. 2004; 29(15):1681–1688

[6] Sofianos DA, Briseño MR, Abrams J, Patel AA. Complications of the lateral transpsoas approach for lumbar interbody arthrodesis: a case series and literature review. Clin Orthop Relat Res. 2012; 470(6):1621–1632

[7] Uribe JS, Arredondo N, Dakwar E, Vale FL. Defining the safe working zones using the minimally invasive lateral retroperitoneal transpsoas approach: an anatomical study. J Neurosurg Spine. 2010; 13(2):260–266

[8] Park DK, Lee MJ, Lin EL, Singh K, An HS, Phillips FM. The relationship of intrapsoas nerves during a transpsoas approach to the lumbar spine: anatomic study. J Spinal Disord Tech. 2010; 23(4):223–228

[9] Benglis DM, Vanni S, Levi AD. An anatomical study of the lumbosacral plexus as related to the minimally invasive transpsoas approach to the lumbar spine. J Neurosurg Spine. 2009; 10(2):139–144

[10] Ozgur BM, Aryan HE, Pimenta L, Taylor WR. Extreme lateral interbody fusion (XLIF): a novel surgical technique for anterior lumbar interbody fusion. Spine J. 2006; 6(4):435–443

[11] Knight RQ, Schwaegler P, Hanscom D, Roh J. Direct lateral lumbar interbody fusion for degenerative conditions: early complication profile. J Spinal Disord Tech. 2009; 22(1):34–37

# 11 Lateral Interbody Cages

*Adam B. Wiggins, Benjamin Khechen, Brittany E. Haws, Jordan A. Guntin, Kaitlyn L. Cardinal, Eric H. Lamoutte, and Kern Singh*

## 11.1 Introduction

Perhaps the most distinguishing characteristic of lateral interbody cages is the larger footprints they afford, in addition to accommodating multiple methods of supplemental fixation.[1,2] The rate of subsidence appears to be lower when wider cages are used,[1,2] as evidenced by lateral interbody cages demonstrating lower rates of subsidence than comparable posterior interbody cages.[1]

## 11.2 Static PEEK Lateral Interbody Cages

**Table 11.1** Globus Medical TransContinental®

| Design | | |
|---|---|---|
| **Cage type** | **Composition** | **Design feature** |
| Static | Polyetheretherketone (PEEK) | Sizable single-graft chamber facilitates bony consolidation |

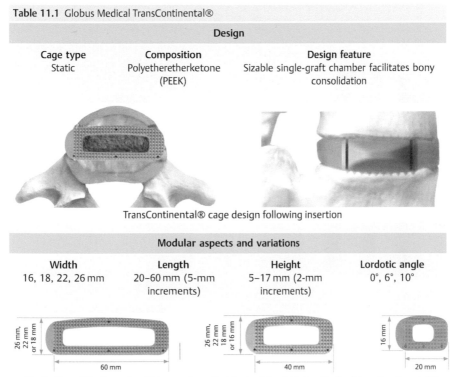

TransContinental® cage design following insertion

| Modular aspects and variations | | | |
|---|---|---|---|
| **Width** | **Length** | **Height** | **Lordotic angle** |
| 16, 18, 22, 26 mm | 20–60 mm (5-mm increments) | 5–17 mm (2-mm increments) | 0°, 6°, 10° |

Illustration of the largest, midsize, and smallest footprints of Globus Medical TransContinental®

**Table 11.1** (*Continued*) Globus Medical TransContinental®

| Procedures |
| --- |
| MIS LLIF |

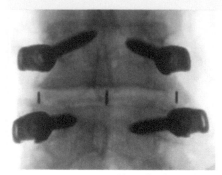 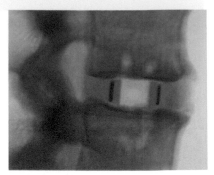

AP and lateral radiographs of Globus Medical TransContinental®

| Supplemental fixation systems |
| --- |
| Globus Medical REVOLVE® posterior stabilization system for MIS |

**Table 11.2** K2 M ALEUTIAN® Lateral Interbody System

| Design | | |
|---|---|---|
| **Cage type**<br>Static | **Composition**<br>Polyetheretherketone<br>(PEEK) | **Design feature**<br>Bulleted nose with circumferential rings<br>designed to grip end plates |

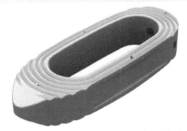

Oblique illustration of ALEUTIAN® Lateral Interbody System

| Modular aspects and variations | | | |
|---|---|---|---|
| **Width**<br>16, 18, 22 mm | **Length**<br>25–60 mm (5-mm<br>increments) | **Height**<br>6, 7, 8–16 mm (2-mm<br>increments) | **Lordotic angle**<br>0°, 8°, 12°, 15° |

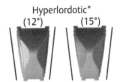

Parallel  Lordotic (8°)  Hyperlordotic* (12°) (15°)

Available sagittal profile options for the ALEUTIAN® Lateral Interbody system

| Procedures |
|---|
| MIS LLIF |
| Radiographs unavailable |

| Supplemental fixation systems |
|---|
| K2 M RAVINE® Lateral Access System |

**Table 11.3** NuVasive CoRoent® Large Oblique (LO) Interbody Cage Device

| Design | | |
|---|---|---|
| **Cage type** | **Composition** | **Design feature** |
| Static | Polyetheretherketone (PEEK) | Designed specifically for oblique placement |

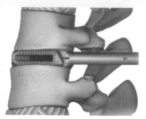 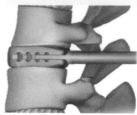

CoRoent® LO placement utilizes the insert (left) and rotate (right) technique

| Modular aspects and variations | | | |
|---|---|---|---|
| **Width** | **Length** | **Height** | **Lordotic angle** |
| 10 mm | 25, 30, 35, 40 mm | 8, 10, 12, 14 mm | 5° |

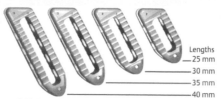

Lengths
— 25 mm
— 30 mm
— 35 mm
— 40 mm

Available length for the CoRoent® LO Interbody Cage Device

**Procedures**

MIS TLIF, MIS LLIF

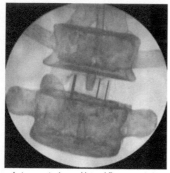 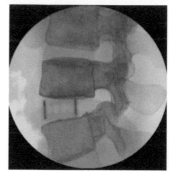

Anteroposterior and lateral fluoroscopic images of NuVasive CoRoent® LO Interbody Cage Device

**Supplemental fixation systems**

NuVasive Reline®, Precept®, or Armada® posterior stabilization systems for MIS

**Table 11.4** RTI Surgical Cross-Fuse® II PEEK VBR/IBF System

| Design | | |
|---|---|---|
| **Cage type** | **Composition** | **Design feature** |
| Static | PEEK-OPTIMA® from Invibio® Biomaterial Solutions | Graft window internal ridges enhance surface area for graft containment and features anatomy matching tooth geometry to minimize device movement |

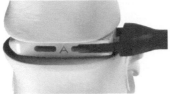 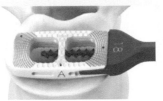

RTI Surgical Cross-Fuse® II cage upon insertion

| Modular aspects and variations | |
|---|---|
| **Widths** | **Lordotic angles** |
| 14, 18, 22, 26 mm | 6° and 12° |

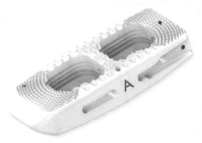

| Procedures |
|---|
| MIS LLIF |

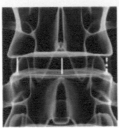 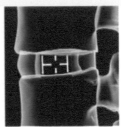

Anteroposterior and lateral radiographic illustrations of RTI Surgical Cross-Fuse® II PEEK VBR/IBF System

| Supplemental fixation systems |
|---|
| RTI Surgical's Streamline® TL or Streamline® MIS Spinal Fixation Systems |

# 11.3 Static Metal Interbody Cages

**Table 11.5** K2 M CASCADIA™ Lateral

| Design | | |
|---|---|---|
| **Cage type** | **Composition** | **Design feature** |
| Static | Titanium | Titanium technology promotes bony integration of the implant |

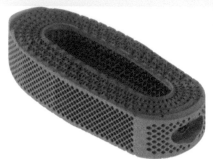

Illustration of the CASCADIA™ Lateral cage design

| Modular aspects and variations | | | |
|---|---|---|---|
| **Width** | **Length** | **Height** | **Lordotic angle** |
| 22 mm | 45–60 mm (5-mm increments) | 8–14 mm (2-mm increments) | 0° and 8° |

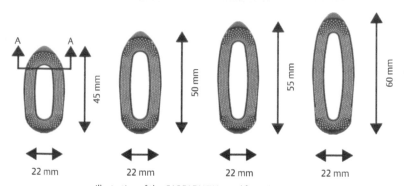

Illustration of the CASCADIA™ Lateral footprint options

| Procedures |
|---|
| MIS LLIF |
| Radiographs unavailable |

| Supplemental fixation systems |
|---|
| K2 M Terra Nova® stabilization system |

# 11.4 Static Mixed Composition Interbody Cages

**Table 11.6** DePuy Synthes COUGAR® LS Lateral Cage System

| Design | | |
|---|---|---|
| **Cage type** | **Composition** | **Design feature** |
| Static | Polyetheretherketone (PEEK)/carbon fiber reinforced polymer (CFRP) | PEEK/CFRP material enhances cage strength |

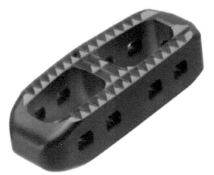

Illustration of the COUGAR® LS Lateral Cage System

| **Width** | **Length** | **Height** | **Lordotic angle** |
|---|---|---|---|
| 15, 18, 21 mm | 30–60 mm (5-mm increments) | 6–16 mm (2-mm increments) | 0°, 7.5° |

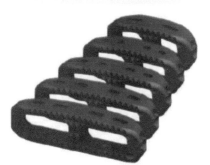

The COUGAR® LS Lateral Cage System is available in several sizes to accommodate for anatomical variations

**Table 11.6** (*Continued*) DePuy Synthes COUGAR® LS Lateral Cage System

| Procedures |
| --- |
| MIS LLIF |

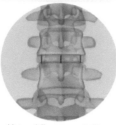 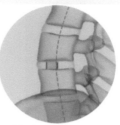

Anteroposterior and lateral fluoroscopic illustrations of DePuy Synthes COUGAR® LS Lateral Cage System

| Supplemental fixation systems |
| --- |
| DePuy Synthes supplemental fixation systems for MIS |

**Table 11.7** Globus Medical TransContinental® titanium plasma spray (TPS)

| Design | | |
|---|---|---|
| **Cage type** | **Composition** | **Design feature** |
| Static | Polyetheretherketone (PEEK) with TPS | Sizable single-graft chamber promotes large fusion mass |

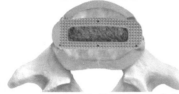 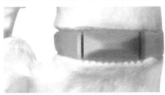

TransContinental® cage design following insertion (PEEK model shown)

| Modular Aspects and Variations | | | |
|---|---|---|---|
| **Width** | **Length** | **Height** | **Lordotic angle** |
| 16, 18, 22, 26 mm | 20–60 mm (5-mm increments) | 5–17 mm (2-mm increments) | 0°, 6°, 10° |

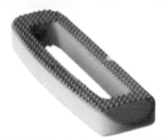

Oblique illustration of TransContinental® with TPS coating

| Procedures |
|---|
| MIS LLIF |

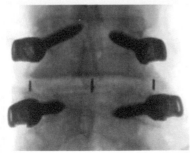 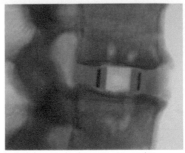

Anteroposterior and lateral fluoroscopic images of Globus Medical TransContinental®

| Supplemental fixation systems |
|---|
| Globus Medical REVOLVE® stabilization system for MIS |

# 11.5 Expandable Interbody Cages

**Table 11.8** Globus Medical CALIBER®-L

| Design | | |
| --- | --- | --- |
| **Cage type**<br>Expandable | **Composition**<br>Titanium with poly-etheretherketone (PEEK) | **Design feature**<br>Coronal taper options allow for a customized fit |

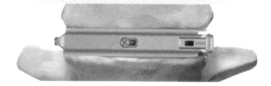

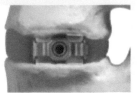

CALIBER®-L cage design following expansion

| Modular aspects and variations | | | |
| --- | --- | --- | --- |
| **Width**<br>16, 18, 22 mm | **Length**<br>25–60 mm | **Height**<br>7–12 mm, with 5-mm expansion | **Lordotic angle**<br>6°, 10°, or 0° |

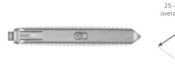
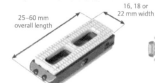
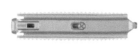

25–60 mm overall length

16, 18 or 22 mm width

Continuous expansion of the CALIBER®-L helps resist migration by optimizing fit

| Procedures |
| --- |
| MIS LLIF |

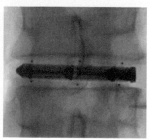
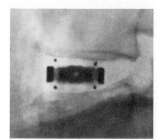

Anteroposterior and lateral radiographs of Globus Medical CALIBER®-L

| Supplemental fixation systems |
| --- |
| Globus Medical REVOLVE® stabilization system |

**Table 11.9** Globus Medical RISE®-L

| Design | | |
|---|---|---|
| **Cage type** | **Composition** | **Design feature** |
| Expandable | Titanium | In situ introduction of allograft maximizes fusion potential |

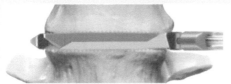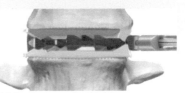

Cage design upon initial insertion (left) and following expansion (right)

| Modular aspects and variations | | | |
|---|---|---|---|
| **Width** | **Length** | **Expansion ranges** | **Lordotic angle** |
| 18 and 22 mm | 40–60 mm (5-mm increments) | 7–17 mm | 0°, 6°, 10° |

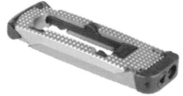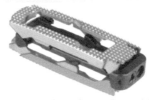

The RISE®-L provides up to 7mm of continuous expansion depending on the model

| Procedures |
|---|
| MIS LLIF |

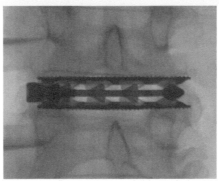

Anteroposterior fluoroscopic image of Globus Medical RISE®-L

| Supplemental fixation systems |
|---|
| Globus Medical REVOLVE® stabilization system |

# References

[1] Pawar A, Hughes A, Girardi F, Sama A, Lebl D, Cammisa F. Lateral lumbar interbody fusion. Asian Spine J. 2015; 9(6):978–983

[2] Kwon B, Kim DH. Lateral lumbar interbody fusion: indications, outcomes, and complications. J Am Acad Orthop Surg. 2016; 24(2):96–105

# 12 Lateral Fixation Systems

*Simon P. Lalehzarian, Benjamin Khechen, Brittany E. Haws, Kaitlyn L. Cardinal, Jordan A. Guntin, Eric H. Lamoutte, and Kern Singh*

## 12.1 Introduction

Vertebral plates are another type of instrumentation used for spinal fixation. Historically, lateral lumbar interbody fusions (LLIFs) were performed as stand-alone procedures.[1] However, stand-alone interbody cages exhibited questionable stability due to limited resistance in vertebral motion.[2][3][4] As such, supplemental fixation has been frequently utilized. However, posterior fixation in this setting requires patient repositioning and may increase the risk of complications and may increase morbidity.[1] Lateral plates can be used in the setting of minimally invasive lateral approaches with the advantage of utilizing the same surgical approach as the interbody cage.[1] This avoids the need for patient repositioning and reduces the risk of additional procedures. These instruments are often composed of a titanium plate with multiple screw slots for fixation to the vertebral body. Occasionally, the plate and screws are integrated with the interbody cage (Chapter 11 Lateral Interbody Cages) or VBR Device (Chapter 13 Vertebral Body Replacement Devices) in order to facilitate hardware placement.[5] Surgical indications are presented in ▶ Table 12.1.

## 12.2 Outcomes

Screw–plate constructs have exhibited successful outcomes in reducing vertebral motion following interbody fusions.[6] Lateral plates have been demonstrated to increase lumbar rigidity in flexion and extension.[6][7] Lateral plates have also been noted to substantially reduce motion in lateral bending and axial rotation.[8] Compared to bilateral pedicle screws (Chapter 3), screw–plate constructs have exhibited similar efficacy in terms of fixation and reducing vertebral motion. Furthermore, the utilization of lateral plates for fixation has been suggested to reduce patient morbidity.[6][9] Previous studies have demonstrated shorter operative times, reduced blood loss, and decreased time under fluoroscopy.[6] Plate instrumentation may also avoid many of the complications associated with posterior fixation, such as iatrogenic neurologic injury.[6]

Table 12.1 Surgical indications for vertebral plates

| Indications |
| --- |
| • Lateral approach spinal fusion |
| • Thoracolumbar procedures |
| • Degenerative disk disease |
| • Spondylolisthesis |
| • Spinal fracture/dislocation |

# 12.3 Lateral Fixation Device Systems

**Table 12.2** Globus Medical InterContinental® LLIF Plate-Spacer System

| Design | |
| --- | --- |
| **Composition** | **Design feature** |
| Titanium and polyetheretherketone (PEEK) | Plate and spacer assembled intraoperatively to minimize disruption to patient anatomy |
| | Two bone screws secure the plate-spacer and compressively load the graft chamber to promote fusion |

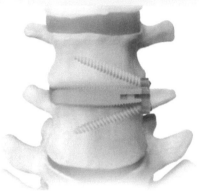

Globus Medical InterContinental® LLIF Plate-Spacer System final construct

| Modular aspects and variations | | | | | |
| --- | --- | --- | --- | --- | --- |
| **Plate-Spacer specifications** | | | | **Screw Specifications** | |
| **Width** | **Lengths** | **Lordotic angle** | **Heights** | **Diameter** | **Lengths** |
| 20 mm | 40–65 mm (5-mm increments) | 0°, 6°, 20°, 25° | 0°, 6°: 8–17 mm 20°, 25°: 11–21 mm | 5.5 mm | 30–55 mm (5-mm increments) |

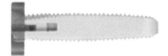

Plate-Spacer implant

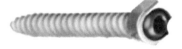

Self-tapping screw

**Table 12.2** (*Continued*) Globus Medical InterContinental® LLIF Plate-Spacer System

| Procedures |
| --- |
| MIS LLIF, MIS corpectomy |

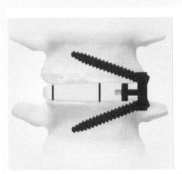 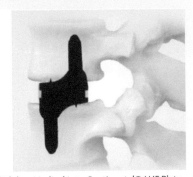

Anteroposterior and lateral radiographic illustrations of Globus Medical InterContinental® LLIF Plate-Spacer System placement

| Supplemental fixation system |
| --- |
| Globus Medical TransContinental® M Spacer System, InterContinental® Plate System, Minimal Access Retractor System |

**Table 12.3** Globus Medical PLYMOUTH® Thoracolumbar Plate System

| Design | | |
|---|---|---|
| **Composition**<br>Titanium | **Design feature**<br>2- and 4-screw plate designs with simple locking set screw to allow visual confirmation | |

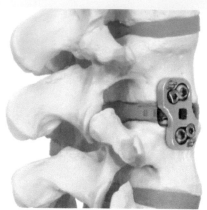

Globus Medical PLYMOUTH® Thoracolumbar Plate System: 2-screw plate final construct

| Modular aspects and variations | | |
|---|---|---|
| **Screw diameter**<br>5.5 and 6.5 mm | **Screw lengths**<br>22–57 mm | **Plate lengths**<br>15–24 mm |

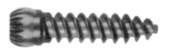

Fixed angle screw                                   2- and 4-screw plates

| Procedures |
|---|
| MIS LLIF, MIS corpectomy |
| Radiographs unavailable |

| Supplemental fixation system |
|---|
| Globus Medical TransContinental® M Spacer System, CALIBER®-L Interbody Systems |

**Table 12.4** K2 M CAYMAN® Minimally Invasive Plate System

| Design | | |
| --- | --- | --- |
| **Composition** | **Design feature** | |
| Titanium | TiFix locking technology enhances plate fixation and promotes stability | |

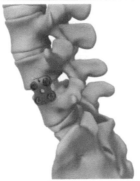

K2M CAYMAN® Minimally Invasive Plate System final construct

| Modular aspects and variations | | |
| --- | --- | --- |
| **Screw diameters** | **Screw lengths** | **Plate lengths** |
| 5 and 5.5 mm | 24–60 mm (4-mm increments) | 8–18 mm (2-mm increments) |

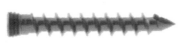

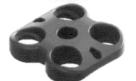

Self-starting screw                                        One-level lateral plate

| Procedures |
| --- |
| MIS LLIF, MIS corpectomy |

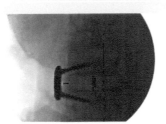
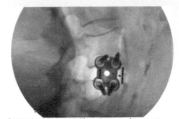

Anteroposterior and lateral fluoroscopic image of K2M CAYMAN® MI Plate System placement

| Supplemental fixation system |
| --- |
| K2 M RAVINE® Lateral Access System, ALEUTIAN® Lateral Interbody System |

**Table 12.5** NuVasive SpheRx® II Anterior System

| Design | |
|---|---|
| **Composition** | **Design feature** |
| Titanium | Multiple staple sizes with 10-mm-long fixation spikes designed to fit unpredictable patient anatomy |

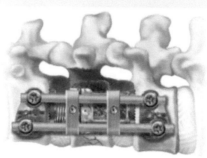

NuVasive SpheRx® II Anterior System final construct

| Modular aspects and variations | | | |
|---|---|---|---|
| **Polyaxial screw specifications** | | **Fixed-screw specifications** | |
| **Diameter** | **Lengths** | **Diameter** | **Lengths** |
| 5.5, 6.5, 7.5 mm | 25–50 mm (5-mm increments) | 5.5, 6.5, 7.5 mm | 25–60 mm (5-mm increments) |

| Procedures |
|---|
| MIS LLIF, MIS corpectomy |
| Radiographs unavailable |

| Supplemental fixation system |
|---|
| NuVasive MaXcess® Access System, XLIF® Expandable VBR System |

**Table 12.6** NuVasive Traverse® Anterior Plate System

| Design | | |
|---|---|---|
| **Composition** | **Design feature** | |
| Titanium | Compression plate utilizes Spiralock® unidirectional locking thread to minimize cross-threading | |
| | Fixed plate utilizes canted coil locking mechanism | |

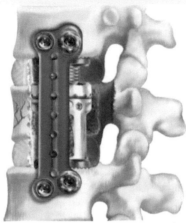

NuVasive Traverse® Anterior Plate System Compression Plate final construct

| Modular aspects and variations | | | |
|---|---|---|---|
| **Screw diameters** | **Screw lengths** | **Compression plate lengths** | **Fixed plate sizes** |
| 5.5 and 6.5 mm | 25–65 mm (5-mm increments) | 45–80 mm (5-mm increments), 85, 95, 105 mm | 15–70 (5-mm increments), 80, 90 mm |

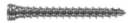

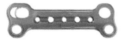

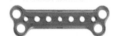

| Bone screw | 2-bolt, 2-screw compression plate | 4-screw fixed plate |
|---|---|---|

**Table 12.6** (*Continued*) NuVasive Traverse® Anterior Plate System

| Procedures |
| --- |
| MIS LLIF and MIS corpectomy |

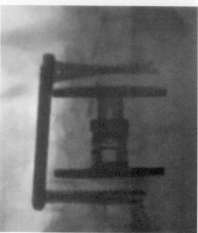

Anteroposterior radiograph of NuVasive Traverse® Anterior Plate System placement

| Supplemental fixation system |
| --- |
| MaXcess® Access System, XLIF® Expandable VBR System |

**Table 12.7** RTI Surgical Lat-Fuse® Lateral Plate System

| Design | |
| --- | --- |
| **Composition** | **Design feature** |
| Titanium | Utilizes expanding sphere locking mechanism that allows for visual confirmation |

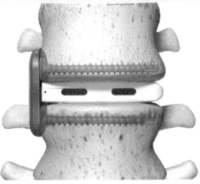

RTI Surgical Lat-Fuse Lateral® Plate System and Cross-Fuse® II PEEK VBR device final construct

| Modular aspects and variations | | |
| --- | --- | --- |
| **Screw diameter** | **Screw lengths** | **Plate lengths** |
| 5.5 and 6.5 mm | 30 mm, 40–70 mm (5-mm increments) | 14–28 mm (2-mm increments) |

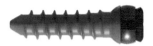

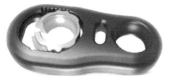

| Self-drilling screw | Lat-fuse lateral plate |
| --- | --- |

| Procedures |
| --- |

MIS LLIF, MIS corpectomy

Radiographs unavailable

**Table 12.8** Zimmer Biomet Timberline® MPF Lateral Modular Plate Fixation System

| Design | |
|---|---|
| **Composition** | **Design feature** |
| Titanium and polyetheretherketone (PEEK) | 1-, 2-, and 4-screw plate designs with single-step lock plate to prevent screw back |

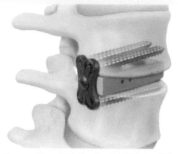
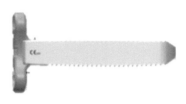

Zimmer Biomet Timberline® MPF Lateral Modular Plate Fixation System final construct and freestanding plate-spacer implant

| Modular aspects and variations | | | | | |
|---|---|---|---|---|---|
| **Plate-spacer specifications** | | | | **Screw specifications** | |
| **Widths** | **Lengths** | **Lordotic angle** | **Heights** | **Diameter** | **Lengths** |
| 18 and 22 mm | 45–60 mm (5-mm increments) | 0°, 8° | 8–14 mm (2-mm increments) | 5.5 and 6 mm | 30–60 mm (5-mm increments) |

| Procedures |
|---|
| MIS LLIF, MIS corpectomy |

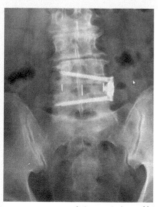
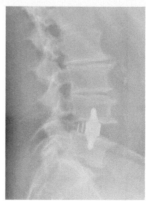

Anteroposterior and lateral radiographs of Timberline® MPF

| Supplemental fixation system |
|---|
| Zimmer Biomet Supplemental Fixation System |

# References

[1] Tzermiadianos MN, Mekhail A, Voronov LI, et al. Enhancing the stability of anterior lumbar interbody fusion: a biomechanical comparison of anterior plate versus posterior transpedicular instrumentation. Spine. 2008; 33(2):E38–E43

[2] Nibu K, Panjabi MM, Oxland T, Cholewicki J. Multidirectional stabilizing potential of BAK interbody spinal fusion system for anterior surgery. J Spinal Disord. 1997; 10(4):357–362

[3] Oxland TR, Hoffer Z, Nydegger T, Rathonyi GC, Nolte LP. A comparative biomechanical investigation of anterior lumbar interbody cages: central and bilateral approaches. J Bone Joint Surg Am. 2000; 82(3):383–393

[4] Heth JA, Hitchon PW, Goel VK, Rogge TN, Drake JS, Torner JC. A biomechanical comparison between anterior and transverse interbody fusion cages. Spine. 2001; 26(12):E261–E267

[5] Cain CM, Schleicher P, Gerlach R, Pflugmacher R, Scholz M, Kandziora F. A new stand-alone anterior lumbar interbody fusion device: biomechanical comparison with established fixation techniques. Spine. 2005; 30(23):2631–2636

[6] Fogel GR, Parikh RD, Ryu SI, Turner AW. Biomechanics of lateral lumbar interbody fusion constructs with lateral and posterior plate fixation: laboratory investigation. J Neurosurg Spine. 2014; 20(3):291–297

[7] Fogel GR, Turner AW, Dooley ZA, Cornwall GB. Biomechanical stability of lateral interbody implants and supplemental fixation in a cadaveric degenerative spondylolisthesis model. Spine. 2014; 39(19):E1138–E1146

[8] Cappuccino A, Cornwall GB, Turner AW, et al. Biomechanical analysis and review of lateral lumbar fusion constructs. Spine. 2010; 35(26) Suppl:S361–S367

[9] Youssef JA, McAfee PC, Patty CA, et al. Minimally invasive surgery: lateral approach interbody fusion: results and review. Spine. 2010; 35(26) Suppl:S302–S311

# 13 Vertebral Body Replacement Devices

*Simon P. Lalehzarian, Benjamin Khechen, Brittany E. Haws, Kaitlyn L. Cardinal, Jordan A. Guntin, Eric H. Lamoutte, and Kern Singh*

## 13.1 Introduction

Corpectomy procedures are utilized in the treatment of vertebral compression fractures (VCFs) secondary to an array of pathologies (▶ Table 13.1).[1,2,3,4,5] Bone grafts such as the tricortical iliac bone crest and fibular strut (▶ Fig. 13.1) had previously been considered the gold standard treatments to fill the space vacated following corpectomy.[6,7,8] Although bone graft options have demonstrated clinical efficacy, their use has declined due to an association with postoperative complications such as donor-site pain, immunological rejection, and risk of pseudarthrosis.[9,10,11,12,13] Several vertebral body replacement (VBR) devices have been developed with the purpose to reduce the morbidities associated with bone graft implants.[9,10,11,14,15]

The surgical approach for minimally invasive lumbar corpectomy procedures is similar to that of the lateral lumbar interbody fusion. To mitigate the risk of postoperative nerve root dysfunction, care should be taken to create surgical access anterior to the psoas. Procedures involving the upper lumbar levels provide greater surgical access due to decreased prominence of psoas at these levels. In comparison, procedures involving the lower lumbar levels afford greater difficulty in positioning the retractor anterior to the psoas. As such, more care should be taken when operating at lower lumbar levels to minimize the risk of postoperative nerve root dysfunction.[16]

### 13.1.1 Vertebral Body Replacement Device Classification

Selection of implant depends on several considerations such as bone quality, location in the spine, and the number of operative levels.[15] To optimize the interface between

**Table 13.1** Criteria for vertebral body replacement

| Indications | Contraindications |
| --- | --- |
| • Spinal tumors | • Cervical procedures |
| • Spinal deformity | • Osteoporosis (≥grade 3) |
| • Spinal infections | • Spondylolisthesis (>grade 2) |
| • Degenerative lumbar disease | • Systemic infection |
| • Thoracolumbar burst fractures | |

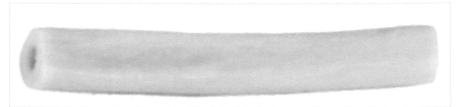

**Fig. 13.1** Fibular strut allograft previously used in corpectomy procedures. (Reproduced with permission of © K2 M Fibular Shaft Bone Graft.)

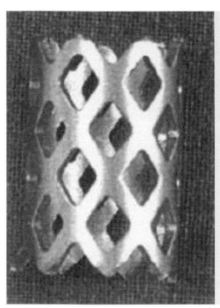

**Fig. 13.2** Previously utilized titanium mesh vertebral body replacement (VBR) implant. (This image is provided courtesy of © DePuy Synthes.)

the vertebral end plates and the VBR device, the implant must feature an adequately sized footprint.[17] Additionally, an effective VBR device should restore physiologic load bearing to the anterior column, and restore both vertebral height and lordosis.[18] VBR cage implants are becoming the preferred treatment for situations in which the area that needs to be occupied following corpectomy is too large for bone graft.[14,15]

## Vertebral Body Replacement Cage Design

The first VBR cages introduced were fixed metal constructs.[19] One of the first designs introduced was the mesh cage (▶ Fig. 13.2), which provided an option when use of bone graft was deemed insufficient.[8] The hollow structure of the mesh cage provides additional area for cancellous bone graft placement to enhance arthrodesis.[8,14,20] Variations in implant length, diameter, and shape (cylindrical, contoured, block) provide improved ability to recreate physiologic vertebral body dimensions and match the sagittal alignment of the prepared vertebral end plates.[21] However, mesh VBR implants have also reported instances of failure, regression of lordosis, and subsidence during follow-up period.[20]

Expandable VBR implants (▶ Fig. 13.3) were developed to improve implant maneuverability and minimize difficulties articulating the implant in the defect space.[22] Particularly in multilevel corpectomy procedures, expandable implants afford the option of a minimally invasive approach by allowing for less challenging, nondistracted insertion through a smaller surgical window.[13]

## Vertebral Body Replacement Cage Composition

Metal and carbon fiber are the two most common materials utilized in VBR implants. Titanium is the most common metal used, and polyetheretherketone (PEEK) is the most common material in carbon fiber constructs. Both compositions have demonstrated

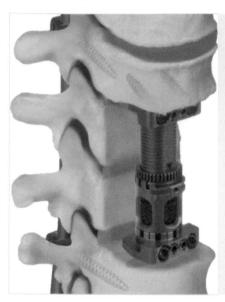

**Fig. 13.3** Illustration depicting an expandable titanium vertebral body replacement (VBR) implant upon insertion. (Image is provided courtesy of © Globus Medical FORTIFY ICorpectomy Spacer System.)

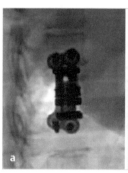
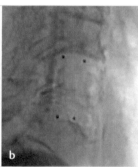

**Fig. 13.4** Lateral fluoroscopy illustrating **(a)** radiopaque titanium and **(b)** radiolucent PEEK expandable VBR implants. (Images are provided courtesy of © Alphatec Spine Novel CP Spinal Spacer System.)

successful outcomes in promoting arthrodesis and restoring vertebral height.[23,24,25,26] However, titanium VBR devices have demonstrated increased stability and reduced micromotion compared to PEEK implants.[27] In comparison, radiolucent PEEK implants allow for improved analysis of arthrodesis and have proven useful in patients with metal allergies (► Fig. 13.4).[24,28,29,30,31] PEEK also provides a stiffness and elasticity comparable to normal patient physiology, which have been thought to enhance the rate of arthrodesis.[29] Varying evidence exists regarding a superior option with regard to fusion rates between titanium and PEEK implants.[25,28,31] As such, further research is necessary to determine the difference in outcomes among material compositions.

## 13.1.2 Efficacy and Outcomes

Through the development of VBRs, corpectomies have been able to provide several advantages over previous surgical treatments for VCFs. Corpectomy procedures have been reported to prevent the loss of long-term vertebral body height correction commonly encountered with cement-only approaches.[32,33,34,35] Eck et al assessed complications and long-term outcomes of 66 patients who received nonexpandable VBR implants following corpectomy.[23] At 2-year follow-up, the average loss of correction of lordosis was less than 1 degree. The authors also reported no instances of cage failure or extrusion. Ender et al performed an investigation of 15 patients with osteoporotic thoracolumbar fractures who received augmentation with expandable titanium mesh cages.[36] At 12 months postoperatively, patients experienced significant improvements in both pain and disability. Furthermore, the degree of vertebral height correction obtained postoperatively was maintained at 12-month follow-up, with no incidences of cage migration or cement-related complications. In another study, Noriega et al utilized an expandable titanium implant in 32 patients with VCFs.[26] At 1-year follow-up, patients experienced significant improvements in pain, narcotics consumption, disability, and quality-of-life metrics. Although VBR devices have demonstrated improved outcomes compared to prior utilized treatments, implant subsidence remains a concern.[37,38] In a study comparing the efficacy of expandable and nonexpandable implants, Lau et al demonstrated that expandable devices were independently associated with higher rates of subsidence compared to nonexpendable implants.[37] Furthermore, the authors reported a greater degree of subsidence associated with expandable implants. In order to effectively determine the ideal implant for corpectomy, additional prospective studies comparing long-term outcomes among VBR devices are required.

# 13.2 Static PEEK VBR Devices

**Table 13.2** Alphatec Spine Novel® CP Spinal Spacer System

| Design | | |
|---|---|---|
| **Type**<br>Static | **Composition**<br>Polyetheretherketone (PEEK) | **Design feature**<br>Toothed end plates and large bone graft windows improve stability and promote bony fusion |

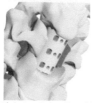 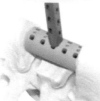

Alphatec Spine Novel® CP Spinal Spacer System upon insertion

| Modular aspects and variations | | |
|---|---|---|
| **Footprint sizes**<br>Small, medium | **Lengths available**<br>10–50 mm (1-mm increments) | **Lordotic angle**<br>5° |

Small

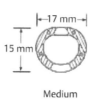

Medium

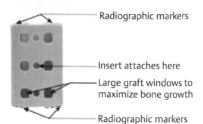

Radiographic markers

Insert attaches here

Large graft windows to maximize bone growth

Radiographic markers

Alphatec Spine Novel® CP Spinal Spacer System footprint dimensions (left) and specifications (right)

| Procedures |
|---|
| MIS corpectomy |

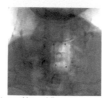 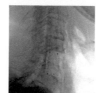

Anteroposterior and lateral fluoroscopic images illustrating Alphatec Spine Novel® CP Spinal Spacer System

| Supplemental fixation system |
|---|
| Alphatec Spine Zodiac® Polyaxial Spinal Fixation System |

**Table 13.3** Globus Medical FORTIFY® I-R Static Corpectomy Spacer System

| Design | | |
|---|---|---|
| **Type** | **Composition** | **Design feature** |
| Static | Polyetheretherketone (PEEK) | Automatic locking system for height stability and preventing collapse |

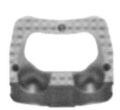

12 × 14 mm

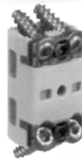

Globus Medical FORTIFY® I-R Static Corpectomy Spacer System footprint (left) and implant (right)

| Modular aspects and variations | | |
|---|---|---|
| **Footprint options** | **Lengths** | **Lordotic angle** |
| 12 × 14 mm | 15–33 mm (2-mm increments) | 0°, 3.5°, 7° |
| **Procedures** | | |
| MIS corpectomy | | |
| Radiographs unavailable | | |
| **Supplemental fixation system** | | |
| Globus Medical CREO MIS™ Spinal Fixation System | | |

**Table 13.4** K2 M SANTORINI® Large Corpectomy Cage System Solid Implant

| Design | | |
| --- | --- | --- |
| **Type** | **Composition** | **Design feature** |
| Static | Polyetheretherketone (PEEK) | Range of heights accommodate smaller anatomy |

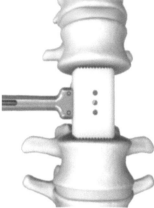

K2M SANTORINI® Large Corpectomy Cage System Solid Implant upon insertion

| Modular aspects and variations | | |
| --- | --- | --- |
| **Footprint sizes** | **Lengths available** | **Lordotic angle** |
| 16 × 20 mm | 22–34 mm | 0° |

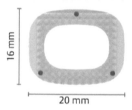 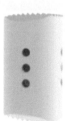

K2M SANTORINI® Large Corpectomy Cage System Solid Implant Footprint Dimensions (left) and cage construct (right)

| Procedures |
| --- |
| MIS corpectomy |
| Radiographs unavailable |

| Supplemental fixation system |
| --- |
| K2 M EVEREST® Posterior Fixation System, K2 M CAYMAN® Lateral Plate Fixation System |

**Table 13.5** RTI Surgical MaxFuse® PEEK VBR System

| Design | | |
| --- | --- | --- |
| **Type** | **Composition** | **Design feature** |
| Static | PEEK-OPTIMA® from Invibio® Biomaterial Solutions | Lateral fenestrations and antimigration teeth allow for improved bony fusion and stability |

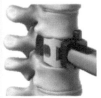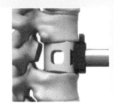

RTI Surgical MaxFuse® Peek VBR System upon insertion

| Modular aspects and variations | | |
| --- | --- | --- |
| **Footprint sizes** | **Length** | **Lordotic angle** |
| 10 × 12, 12 × 14, 14.5 × 17 mm | 12–46 mm (2-mm increments), 47–65 mm (3-mm increments) | 8°, 12°, 16° |

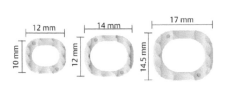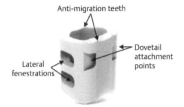

RTI Surgical MaxFuse® PEEK VBR System footprint dimensions (left) and specifications (right)

| Procedures |
| --- |
| MIS corpectomy |
| Radiographs unavailable |

| Supplemental fixation system |
| --- |
| RTI Surgical's Streamline® TL or Streamline® MIS Spinal Fixation System |

## 13.3 Static Metal VBR Devices

Table 13.6 K2 M CAPRI® Small 3D Static Corpectomy Cage System

| Design | | |
|---|---|---|
| **Type** | **Composition** | **Design feature** |
| Static | Titanium | Pore channels from end plate to end plate enhance bony ingrowth |

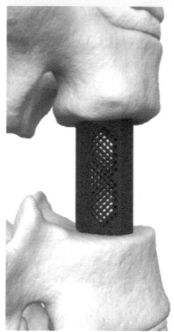

K2M CAPRI® Small 3D Static Corpectomy Cage System upon insertion

| Modular aspects and variations | | |
|---|---|---|
| **Footprint sizes** | **Lengths available** | **Lordotic angle** |
| 12 × 14, 13 × 16 mm | 12–50 mm | 7° |

| 12 × 14 mm | 13 × 16 mm | |

K2M CAPRI® Small 3D Static Corpectomy Cage System Footprint superior view (left and middle) and sagittal view (right)

**Table 13.6** (*Continued*) K2 M CAPRI® Small 3D Static Corpectomy Cage System

| Procedures |
| --- |
| MIS corpectomy |
| Radiographs unavailable |

| Supplemental fixation system |
| --- |
| K2 M Everest® Posterior Fixation System, K2 M CAYMAN® Lateral Plate Fixation System |

**Table 13.7** NuVasive X-CORE® 2 Static VBR

| Design | | |
| --- | --- | --- |
| **Type** | **Composition** | **Implant sizes** |
| Static | Titanium | 16-mm diameter: 12-, 14-mm lengths |
| | | 18-, 22-mm diameter: 16-, 18-mm lengths |

14 mm　　　　　16 mm　　　　　18 mm

NuVasive X-CORE® 2 Static implants of different core diameters and lengths

| Procedures |
| --- |
| MIS corpectomy |
| Radiographs unavailable |

| Supplemental fixation system |
| --- |
| NuVasive XLIF® Decade Plus Lateral Plate System |

# 13.4 Expandable Carbon Fiber VBR Devices

**Table 13.8** DePuy Synthes Spine XRL® Vertebral Body Replacement Device

| Design | | |
|---|---|---|
| **Type**<br>Expandable | **Composition**<br>Polyetheretherketone<br>(PEEK) | **Design feature**<br>Octagonal central body permits various<br>approach options<br>Self-locking expansion mechanism |

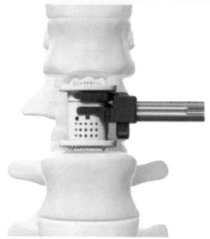

DePuy Synthes Spine XRL® Vertebral Body Replacement Device upon insertion using spreader

| Modular aspects and variations | | | |
|---|---|---|---|
| **Diameter** | **Footprint options** | **Lengths** | **Lordotic angle** |
| 21 mm | 21 × 24, 26 × 30 mm<br>21-mm circumference | 32–142 mm<br>22–36 mm | −10°, −5°, 0°, 5°, 10°,<br>15° |
| 27 mm | 28 × 33, 30 × 40 mm<br>27-mm circumference | 33–145 mm<br>23–37 mm | 0°, 5°, 10°, 15°, 20° |

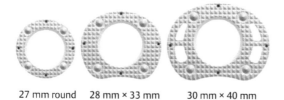 

27 mm round   28 mm × 33 mm   30 mm × 40 mm         27 mm

DePuy Synthes Spine XRL® Vertebral Body Replacement Device large modular (left) and large integrated (right) footprints

**Table 13.8** (*Continued*) DePuy Synthes Spine XRL® Vertebral Body Replacement Device

| Procedures |
| --- |
| MIS corpectomy |
| Radiographs unavailable |
| **Supplemental fixation system** |
| DePuy Synthes USS System including MATRIX Pedicle® Screw System, PANGEA® Pedicle Screw System, and TSLP Locking Plate System |

**Table 13.9** Globus Medical FORTIFY® I-R Expandable Corpectomy Spacer System

| Design | | |
| --- | --- | --- |
| Type | Composition | Design feature |
| Expandable | Polyetheretherketone (PEEK) | Automatic locking system for height stability and preventing collapse |

| Modular aspects and variations | | | |
| --- | --- | --- | --- |
| Diameter | Footprint options | Lengths | Lordotic angle |
| 14 mm | 14 × 14 mm, 14 × 16 mm | 25–97 mm | 0°, 3.5°, 7° |

 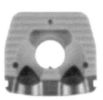 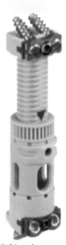

14 × 14 mm    14 × 16 mm

Globus Medical FORTIFY® I- R Expandable Corpectomy Spacer System Footprints (left) and upon expansion (right)

| Procedures |
| --- |
| MIS corpectomy |
| Radiographs unavailable |

| Supplemental fixation system |
| --- |
| Globus Medical Lateral Fixation Systems |

**Table 13.10** K2 M SANTORINI® Large Corpectomy Cage System Expandable Implant

| Design | | |
|---|---|---|
| **Type** | **Composition** | **Design feature** |
| Expandable | Polyetheretherketone (PEEK) | Locking clip design secures expandable cage at desired height |

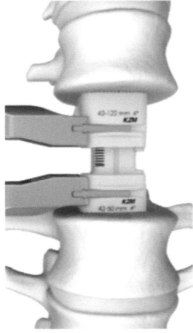

K2M SANTORINI® Large Corpectomy Cage System Expandable Implant upon insertion

| Modular aspects and variations | | |
|---|---|---|
| **Footprint sizes** | **Lengths** | **Lordotic angle** |
| 16 × 20 mm | 36–58 mm | 0°, 4°, 8°, 12°, 16° |
| 21 × 25 mm | 42–98 mm | 0°, 4°, 8°, 12°, 16° |

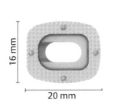 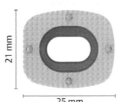

K2M SANTORINI® Large Corpectomy Cage System Expandable Implant Footprint Dimensions

**Table 13.10** (*Continued*) K2 M SANTORINI® Large Corpectomy Cage System Expandable Implant

| Procedures |
| --- |
| MIS corpectomy |
| Radiographs unavailable |
| **Supplemental fixation system** |
| K2 M EVEREST® Posterior Fixation System, K2 M CAYMAN® Lateral Plate Fixation System |

# 13.5 Expandable Metal VBR Devices

**Table 13.11** Globus Medical FORTIFY® I Corpectomy Spacer System

| Design | | |
|---|---|---|
| **Type** | **Composition** | **Design feature** |
| Expandable | Titanium | Automatic locking system for height stability and preventing collapse |

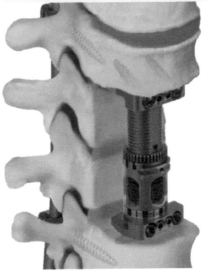

Titanium core implant from Globus Medical FORTIFY® I Corpectomy Spacer System after insertion

| Modular aspects and variations | | | |
|---|---|---|---|
| **Diameter** | **Footprint options** | **Lengths** | **Lordotic angle** |
| 12 mm | 12 × 14, 14 × 16 mm | 23–97 mm | 0°, 3.5°, 7° |
| 20 mm | 21 × 23, 25 × 30 mm 22 × 40, 22 × 45, 22 × 50 mm | 32–132 mm 30–129 mm | 0°, 4°, 8°, 12°, 16° 0°, 4°, 8°, 12° |

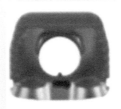 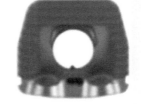

12 × 14 mm          14 × 16 mm

Globus Medical FORTIFY® I Corpectomy Spacer System footprints

**Table 13.11** (*Continued*) Globus Medical FORTIFY® I Corpectomy Spacer System

| Procedures |
| --- |
| MIS corpectomy |
| Radiographs unavailable |

| Supplemental fixation system |
| --- |
| Globus Medical Lateral Fixation System |

**Table 13.12** K2 M CAPRI® Corpectomy Cage System

| Design | | |
|---|---|---|
| **Type** | **Composition** | **Design feature** |
| Expandable | Titanium and cobalt chrome | Allows for in-situ height expansion and end plate angulation |

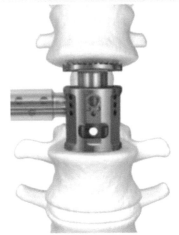

K2M CAPRI® Corpectomy Cage System upon insertion and expansion

| Modular aspects and variations | | | |
|---|---|---|---|
| **Footprint sizes** | **Lengths** | **Adjustable end plate angle** | **Lordotic angle** |
| 17 × 22, 21 × 25 mm | 23–74 mm | −20° to 20° | 0° |
| 24 × 30, 28 × 36 mm | 30–122 mm | −20° to 20° | 0°, 10°, 20° |

17 × 22 mm   21 × 25 mm   24 × 30 mm   28 × 36 mm

K2M CAPRI® Corpectomy Cage System Footprint Dimensions (left) and adjustable angulation (right)

| Procedures |
|---|
| MIS corpectomy |
| Radiographs unavailable |

| Supplemental fixation system |
|---|
| K2 M EVEREST® Posterior Fixation System, K2 M CAYMAN® Lateral Plate Fixation System |

**Table 13.13** NuVasive X-CORE® Expandable VBR

| Design | | |
|---|---|---|
| **Type** | **Composition** | **Design feature** |
| Expandable | Titanium | Expandable, angulating end caps enhance implant stability |

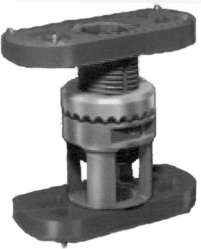

X-CORE® Expandable Implant Insertion during XLIF Corpectomy Procedure

| Modular aspects and variations | | | |
|---|---|---|---|
| **Core diameter** | **Footprint sizes** | **Lengths** | **Lordotic angle** |
| 18 mm | 22-, 26-mm circumference, 18 × 30, 18 × 40, 18 × 50 mm | 20–75 mm | −4°, 0°, 4°, 8° |
| 22 mm | 30-mm circumference, 22 × 40, 22 × 50, 22 × 60 mm | 20–75 mm | 0°, 4°, 8°, 12° |

| Procedures |
|---|
| MIS corpectomy |

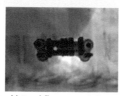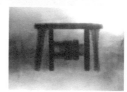

Anteroposterior and lateral fluoroscopic images of NuVasive X-CORE® Expandable VBR placement (with Traverse® Plate)

| Supplemental fixation system |
|---|
| NuVasive MaXcess® Access System, Traverse® Anterior Plate System, SpheRx® II Anterior Dual Rod System |

**Table 13.14** NuVasive X-CORE® 2 Expandable VBR

| Design | | |
|---|---|---|
| **Type** | **Composition** | **Design feature** |
| Expandable | Titanium | Expandable, angulating end caps enhance implant stability |

NuVasive X-CORE® 2 Expandable VBR upon Insertion and Expansion (left) and final placement (right)

| Modular aspects and variations | | | |
|---|---|---|---|
| **Core diameter** | **Footprint sizes** | **Lengths** | **Lordotic angle** |
| 16 mm | 16-, 18-mm circumference, 16 × 30, 16 × 40 mm | 16–75 mm | –4°, 0°, 4° |
| 18 mm | 18-, 22-, 26-mm circumference, 18 × 30, 18 × 40, 18 × 50 mm 22 × 30, 22 × 40, 22 × 50, 22 × 60 mm | 20–121 mm | –4°, 0°, 4°, 8° 0°, 4°, 8°, 12° |
| 22 mm | 22-, 26-, 30-mm circumference, 22 × 40, 22 × 50, 22 × 60 mm | 20–121 mm | 0°, 4°, 8°, 12° |

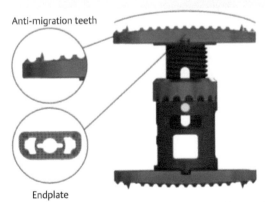

Anti-migration teeth

Endplate

NuVasive X-CORE® 2 Expandable 18-mm implant with design features showcased

**Table 13.14** *(Continued)* NuVasive X-CORE® 2 Expandable VBR

| Procedures |
| --- |
| MIS corpectomy |

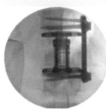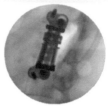

Anteroposterior and lateral fluoroscopic images illustrating NuVasive X-CORE® 2 Expandable VBR placement

| Supplemental fixation system |
| --- |
| NuVasive XLIF Decade Plus Plate System |

# References

[1] Cotler HB, Cotler JM, Stoloff A, et al. The use of autografts for vertebral body replacement of the thoracic and lumbar spine. Spine. 1985; 10(8):748–756

[2] Finkelstein JA, Chapman JR, Mirza S. Anterior cortical allograft in thoracolumbar fractures. J Spinal Disord. 1999; 12(5):424–429

[3] Hussein AA, El-Karef E, Hafez M. Reconstructive surgery in spinal tumours. Eur J Surg Oncol. 2001; 27(2):196–199

[4] Streitz W, Brown JC, Bonnett CA. Anterior fibular strut grafting in the treatment of kyphosis. Clin Orthop Relat Res. 1977(128):140–148

[5] Theologis AA, Tabaraee E, Toogood P, et al. Anterior corpectomy via the mini-open, extreme lateral, transpsoas approach combined with short-segment posterior fixation for single-level traumatic lumbar burst fractures: analysis of health-related quality of life outcomes and patient satisfaction. J Neurosurg Spine. 2016; 24(1):60–68

[6] Kurz LT, Garfin SR, Booth RE, Jr. Harvesting autogenous iliac bone grafts. A review of complications and techniques. Spine. 1989; 14(12):1324–1331

[7] Sacks S. Anterior interbody fusion of the lumbar spine. Indications and results in 200 cases. Clin Orthop Relat Res. 1966; 44(44):163–170

[8] Karaeminogullari O, Tezer M, Ozturk C, Bilen FE, Talu U, Hamzaoglu A. Radiological analysis of titanium mesh cages used after corpectomy in the thoracic and lumbar spine: minimum 3 years' follow-up. Acta Orthop Belg. 2005; 71(6):726–731

[9] An HS, Lynch K, Toth J. Prospective comparison of autograft vs. allograft for adult posterolateral lumbar spine fusion: differences among freeze-dried, frozen, and mixed grafts. J Spinal Disord. 1995; 8(2):131–135

[10] Nemzek JA, Arnoczky SP, Swenson CL. Retroviral transmission in bone allotransplantation. The effects of tissue processing. Clin Orthop Relat Res. 1996(324):275–282

[11] Sandhu HS, Boden SD. Biologic enhancement of spinal fusion. Orthop Clin North Am. 1998; 29(4):621–631

[12] Lin PM. Posterior lumbar interbody fusion technique: complications and pitfalls. Clin Orthop Relat Res. 1985(193):90–102

[13] Pflugmacher R, Schleicher P, Schaefer J, et al. Biomechanical comparison of expandable cages for vertebral body replacement in the thoracolumbar spine. Spine. 2004; 29(13):1413–1419

[14] Robertson PA, Rawlinson HJ, Hadlow AT. Radiologic stability of titanium mesh cages for anterior spinal reconstruction following thoracolumbar corpectomy. J Spinal Disord Tech. 2004; 17(1):44–52

[15] Vaccaro AR, Cirello J. The use of allograft bone and cages in fractures of the cervical, thoracic, and lumbar spine. Clin Orthop Relat Res. 2002; 394(394):19–26

[16] Singh K, Vaccaro AR. Pocket Atlas of Spine Surgery. New York, NY: Thieme; 2012

[17] Steffen T, Tsantrizos A, Fruth I, Aebi M. Cages: designs and concepts. Eur Spine J. 2000; 9 Suppl 1:S89–S94

[18] Tsantrizos A, Andreou A, Aebi M, Steffen T. Biomechanical stability of five stand-alone anterior lumbar inter-body fusion constructs. Eur Spine J. 2000; 9(1):14–22

[19] Bagby GW. Arthrodesis by the distraction-compression method using a stainless steel implant. Orthopedics. 1988; 11(6):931–934

[20] Zahra B, Jodoin A, Maurais G, Parent S, Mac-Thiong JM. Treatment of thoracolumbar burst fractures by means of anterior fusion and cage. J Spinal Disord Tech. 2012; 25(1):30–37

[21] Dvorak MF, Kwon BK, Fisher CG, Eiserloh HL, III, Boyd M, Wing PC. Effectiveness of titanium mesh cylindrical cages in anterior column reconstruction after thoracic and lumbar vertebral body resection. Spine. 2003; 28(9):902–908

[22] Kandziora F, Pflugmacher R, Schaefer J, et al. Biomechanical comparison of expandable cages for vertebral body replacement in the cervical spine. J Neurosurg. 2003; 99(1) Suppl:91–97

[23] Eck KR, Bridwell KH, Ungacta FF, Lapp MA, Lenke LG, Riew KD. Analysis of titanium mesh cages in adults with minimum two-year follow-up. Spine. 2000; 25(18):2407–2415

[24] Ferguson SJ, Visser JM, Polikeit A. The long-term mechanical integrity of non-reinforced PEEK-OPTIMA polymer for demanding spinal applications: experimental and finite-element analysis. Eur Spine J. 2006; 15(2):149–156

[25] Nemoto O, Asazuma T, Yato Y, Imabayashi H, Yasuoka H, Fujikawa A. Comparison of fusion rates following transforaminal lumbar interbody fusion using polyetheretherketone cages or titanium cages with transpedicular instrumentation. Eur Spine J. 2014; 23(10):2150–2155

[26] Noriega D, Krüger A, Ardura F, et al. Clinical outcome after the use of a new craniocaudal expandable implant for vertebral compression fracture treatment: one year results from a prospective multicentric study. BioMed Res Int. 2015; 2015:927813

[27] Weiner BK, Fraser RD. Spine update lumbar interbody cages. Spine. 1998; 23(5):634–640

[28] Tanida S, Fujibayashi S, Otsuki B, et al. Vertebral endplate cyst as a predictor of nonunion after lumbar inter-body fusion: comparison of titanium and polyetheretherketone cages. Spine. 2016; 41(20):E1216–E1222

[29] Vadapalli S, Sairyo K, Goel VK, et al. Biomechanical rationale for using polyetheretherketone (PEEK) spacers for lumbar interbody fusion: a finite element study. Spine. 2006; 31(26):E992–E998

[30] Toth JM, Wang M, Estes BT, Scifert JL, Seim HB, III, Turner AS. Polyetheretherketone as a biomaterial for spinal applications. Biomaterials. 2006; 27(3):324–334

[31] Cabraja M, Oezdemir S, Koeppen D, Kroppenstedt S. Anterior cervical discectomy and fusion: comparison of titanium and polyetheretherketone cages. BMC Musculoskelet Disord. 2012; 13:172

[32] Heini PF, Teuscher R. Vertebral body stenting / stentoplasty. Swiss Med Wkly. 2012; 142:w13658

[33] Feltes C, Fountas KN, Machinis T, et al. Immediate and early postoperative pain relief after kyphoplasty without significant restoration of vertebral body height in acute osteoporotic vertebral fractures. Neurosurg Focus. 2005; 18(3):e5

[34] Ishiguro S, Kasai Y, Sudo A, Iida K, Uchida A. Percutaneous vertebroplasty for osteoporotic compression fractures using calcium phosphate cement. J Orthop Surg (Hong Kong). 2010; 18(3):346–351

[35] Rotter R, Martin H, Fuerderer S, et al. Vertebral body stenting: a new method for vertebral augmentation versus kyphoplasty. Eur Spine J. 2010; 19(6):916–923

[36] Ender SA, Eschler A, Ender M, Merk HR, Kayser R. Fracture care using percutaneously applied titanium mesh cages (OsseoFix®) for unstable osteoporotic thoracolumbar burst fractures is able to reduce cement-associated complications–results after 12 months. J Orthop Surg Res. 2015; 10:175

[37] Lau D, Song Y, Guan Z, La Marca F, Park P. Radiological outcomes of static vs expandable titanium cages after corpectomy: a retrospective cohort analysis of subsidence. Neurosurgery. 2013; 72(4):529–539, discussion 528–529

[38] Chen Y, Chen D, Guo Y, et al. Subsidence of titanium mesh cage: a study based on 300 cases. J Spinal Disord Tech. 2008; 21(7):489–492

# Part III

## Other

14 Percutaneous Cement
   Augmentation Systems   *180*

15 Biologics   *191*

16 Surgical Navigation
   Systems   *218*

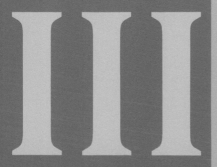

# 14 Percutaneous Cement Augmentation Systems

*Kaitlyn L. Cardinal, Benjamin Khechen, Brittany E. Haws, Jordan A. Guntin, Sravisht Iyer, and Kern Singh*

## 14.1 Introduction

Vertebral compression fractures (VCFs) can result from complications associated with osteoporosis, spinal trauma, or vertebral metastases (▶ Fig. 14.1).[1,2] Osteoporotic VCFs are the most prevalent, with an estimated incidence of 1.4 million per year.[3] VCFs are associated with significant morbidity, including functional limitations, significant pain, and kyphotic deformity.[4,5] Although nonoperative therapy remains the first-line treatment, surgical correction is indicated in cases of uncontrolled pain or progressive deformity.[2] Minimally invasive approaches to VCFs involve percutaneous vertebroplasty or kyphoplasty, with cement augmentation of the vertebral body. Vertebral body cement augmentation is associated with the benefits of improved pain control and may help correct angular deformity.

### 14.1.1 Components

Both vertebroplasty and kyphoplasty are performed under biplanar fluoroscopic guidance. In both procedures, a cannulated trocar is introduced into the vertebral body in conjunction with a spinal needle inserted via a transpedicular route.[6] Trocars can be inserted either unilaterally or bilaterally, depending on the location of the compression deformity and the practitioner's preference. These trocars can accommodate supplementary equipment, including biopsy needles to produce specimens for oncologic testing and drills for removal of bone to create a space for balloon insertion.

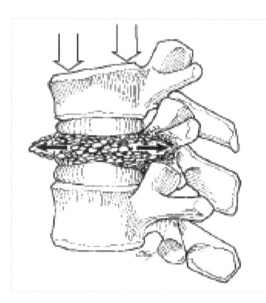

**Fig. 14.1** Depiction of a vertebral compression fracture with associated forces. (Adapted from Baaj AA, Mummaneni PV, Uribe JS, Vaccaro AR, Greenberg MS. Handbook of Spine Surgery; New York, NY: Thieme; 2012.)

In kyphoplasty, orthopaedic balloons are inserted through the trocars into the vertebral body. These balloons are inflated under pressure within the vertebral body, helping create a potential space for cement insertion.[7] The balloons are typically radiopaque and their inflation can be monitored via fluoroscopic guidance. In vertebroplasty, pressurized cement is inserted through the trocar without using a balloon dilator. Shen et al compared the efficacy of kyphoplasty using a vertebral dilator and balloon kyphoplasty to treat osteoporotic thoracolumbar compression fractures.[8] The authors reported postoperative change in the lordosis was significantly greater in the dilator kyphoplasty group than in the balloon kyphoplasty group (−9.51 vs. −7.78 degrees, $p < 0.001$). These findings suggested the vertebral dilator kyphoplasty allows for greater correction of lordotic angle; however, additional prospective studies are required to draw conclusions regarding long-term clinical efficacy.

In both vertebroplasty and kyphoplasty, bone cement is injected through the trocar into the vertebral body. The cement fills the potential space within the vertebral body and provides mechanical support after setting. The bone cement is most commonly comprised of polymethyl methacrylate (PMMA) mixed with barium sulfate. PMMA is a cement polymer that is widely used in orthopaedics due to its biocompatibility and ability to harden quickly.[9] Before injection, PMMA bone cement is mixed with a contrast agent such as barium sulfate, so its introduction into the vertebral body can be fluoroscopically monitored (▶ Fig. 14.2).[7]

## 14.1.2 Outcomes

Multiple level I studies and meta-analyses have been performed with the purpose of analyzing the differences in postoperative outcomes between VCF treatment modalities.[10,11,12] Klazen et al performed a prospective, randomized controlled trial (RCT) of 202 patients undergoing either percutaneous vertebroplasty or conservative management for acute VCFs with Visual Analog Scale (VAS) pain ratings greater than 5.[12] The authors demonstrated that patients receiving cement augmentation had significantly greater pain relief at 1 month and 1 year posttreatment compared to the conservative management group. Furthermore, from a cost perspective, it was noted that cement augmentation was a cost-effective modality when a cutoff of €30,000/quality-adjusted life year (QALY) was used. Farrokhi et al performed a similar prospective RCT with 82 patients undergoing treatment for acute osteoporotic VCF with percutaneous vertebroplasty or conservative management.[11] The patients receiving percutaneous

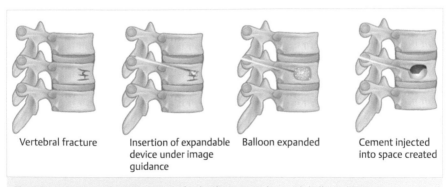

Vertebral fracture — Insertion of expandable device under image guidance — Balloon expanded — Cement injected into space created

**Fig. 14.2** Depiction of a percutaneous kyphoplasty procedure with balloon dilation.

vertebroplasty not only had significantly greater improvements in pain up to 6 months postoperatively but also had greater improvements in disability as measured by the Oswestry Disability Index (ODI) up to 36 months posttreatment. Additionally, the incidence of subsequent vertebral fracture was lower in the cement augmentation group compared to the conservative group (2.2 vs. 13.3%). Using a meta-analysis, Zhao et al compared the efficacy and safety of vertebroplasty, kyphoplasty, and conservative treatment.[13] The authors reported patients who underwent vertebroplasty experienced the greatest pain relief. However, kyphoplasty was the most effective in improving daily function and quality of life. The study also demonstrated that patients who underwent kyphoplasty experienced the lowest incidence of new fractures.

## 14.1.3 Complications

While promising data exists regarding the utility of percutaneous cement augmentation for improvement in clinical outcomes, the technique is not devoid of complications. The most prominent complication is extravasation of cement out of the vertebral body, with reported incidences ranging from 5.0 to 76.83% depending upon the detection modality used.[14,15,16,17,18,19] Although the incidence of cement leakage can be high, most cases are asymptomatic and require no further treatment. While symptomatic cases are rare, they can have significant morbidity and must be managed carefully.[20] Sequelae from symptomatic leakages can include pulmonary embolism, venous embolism leading to cardiovascular collapse, neurologic deficits from spinal stenosis, and adjacent level vertebral fracture.[14,15,16,21,22,23,24] Compared to kyphoplasty, vertebroplasty is associated with a higher incidence of extravasation-related complications as there are higher intraosseous pressures during cement insertion.[14,17,24]

A current trend and recent area of interest within the literature has been the use of unilateral approaches to percutaneous cement augmentation. Published investigations comparing unilateral and bilateral procedures have been supportive of the utility of a unilateral approach, demonstrating similar clinical and radiographic outcomes with distinct perioperative advantages.[25,26,27,28] For example, Yan et al conducted a prospective study of 316 patients with single-level osteoporotic VCFs treated with either unilateral or bilateral percutaneous balloon kyphoplasty.[25] In regard to perioperative factors, the unilateral approach was associated with lower cement volume delivery, shorter operative times, and a reduced radiation dose compared to the bilateral approach. Clinically, both groups demonstrated similar improvements in pain and quality-of-life metrics at final follow-up of at least 24 months postoperatively. Radiographically, both groups had similar improvements in vertebral body height, while the unilateral group had greater kyphotic angle reduction compared to the bilateral group. Total costs were also similar for both groups, taking into account operating room costs, instrument costs, and surgeon's fees. While these investigations suggest the possible superiority of unilateral cement augmentation approaches over bilateral approaches, further investigation is still required to make any definitive conclusions.

# 14.2 Percutaneous Cement Augmentation Systems

**Table 14.1** Benvenue Medical Kiva® Vertebral Compression Fracture Treatment System

| Design |
| --- |
| **Specifications** |
| Implant designed as a mechanical support structure to contain and direct flow of cement |
| Flexible implant made from PEEK-OPTIMA® |

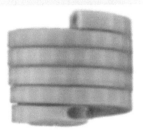

Kiva® VCF Treatment System features a continuous loop (5 total) for cement delivery

| Modular aspects and variations | | |
| --- | --- | --- |
| **Bone access needle** | **Implant** | **Deployment handle** |
| Diamond trocar tip | 20 × 15 mm | Ability to select right or left |
| Bevel tip | | access |

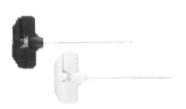

Diamond access trocar tip (blue) and bevel tip (white)

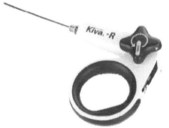

Kiva® deployment handle contains coil and implant

| Procedures |
| --- |
| Percutaneous vertebral compression fracture |

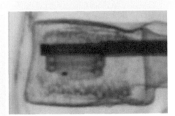 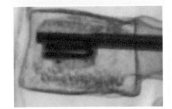

Lateral fluoroscopic images of Benvenue Medical Kiva® coil insertion (left) and cement deployment (right)

**Table 14.2** DePuy Synthes SYNFLATE™ Vertebral Balloon

| Design |
| --- |

### Specifications

Shaft marker on insertion device permits proper advancement into cannula and vertebral body
Inflation system to be filled with liquid contrast medium

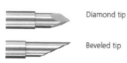

Diamond tip

Beveled tip

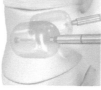

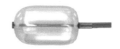

| Different access trocars available | Balloon inserted into vertebral body | Inferior port on insertion device allows for stiffening wire insertion |
| --- | --- | --- |

| Modular aspects and variations | | | |
| --- | --- | --- | --- |
| **Type** | **Small** | **Medium** | **Large** |
| **Length** | 10–18.1 mm | 15 mm | 20 mm |
| **Maximum length** | 18.1 mm | 23.3 mm | 28.9 mm |
| **Diameter** | 16.3 mm | 16.3 mm | 16.3 mm |
| **Maximum volume** | 4.0 mL | 5.0 mL | 6.0 mL |
| **Maximum inflation pressure** | 30 atm (440 psi) | 30 atm (440 psi) | 30 atm (440 psi) |

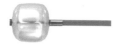
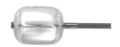

| Small | Medium | Large |
| --- | --- | --- |

| Procedures |
| --- |

Kyphoplasty

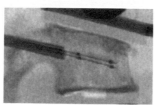
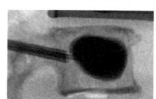

Lateral fluoroscopic images of DePuy Synthes Synflate Balloon insertion

**Table 14.3** DePuy Synthes Vertebral Body Balloon (VBB)

| Design |
|--------|

**Specifications**

Balloon used with cleared spinal polymethylmethacrylate bone cements

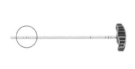 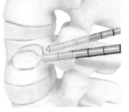 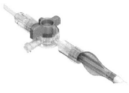

| Insertion device has 3 grooves near distal tip corresponding to sizes of balloons | Balloons being inserted into vertebrae | Three-way stopcock allows for an alternative method of system inflation |
|---|---|---|

| Modular aspects and variations | | | |
|---|---|---|---|
| Type | Small | Medium | Large |
| Preinflated length | 22 mm | 27 mm | 31 mm |
| Maximum diameter | 15 mm | 17 mm | 17 mm |
| Maximum volume | 4.0 mL | 4.5 mL | 5.0 mL |
| Maximum pressure inflation | 30 atm | 30 atm | 30 atm |

| Procedures |
|------------|

Kyphoplasty

Radiographs unavailable

**Table 14.4** DePuy Synthes VERTECEM® Bone Cement

| Design | | |
|---|---|---|
| **Bone cement mixing kit I/II**<br>10% hydroxyapatite<br>Enhanced visibility under fluoroscopy | **Side opening needles**<br>Options for wire or trocar access<br>Beveled and diamond needle | **Syringes**<br>Wide, integrated wings and reinforced syringe pistons |
| 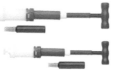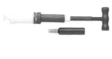<br>Mixing kits are ready to inject after mixing | 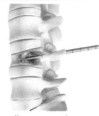<br>Illustration of cement insertion | <br>Syringes provide leverage, rigidity, and tactile feedback |

| Modular aspects and variations | | | | |
|---|---|---|---|---|
| **Gauge** | **Diameter** | **Empty space** | **Tip** | **Extra access** |
| 8 | 4.2 mm | 1.5 mL | Diamond | Guidewire, trocar |
| 10 | 3.4 mm | 0.7 mL | Diamond | Guidewire, trocar |
| 10 | 3.4 mm | 0.7 mL | Beveled | Trocar |
| 12 | 2.7 mm | 0.4 mL | Diamond | Trocar |
| 12 | 2.7 mm | 0.4 mL | Beveled | Trocar |

| Procedures |
|---|
| Vertebroplasty |

Radiographs unavailable

**Table 14.5** Globus Medical AFFIRM® Curved Vertebral Compression Fracture System

| Design |
|---|

**Specifications**
Fully adjustable expanding scraper easily cuts through bone to create specialized cavities
Quad, bevel, and trocar tips available for a variety of instruments
polymethyl methacrylate (PMMA) cement with 28% barium sulfate in 20 or 40 g

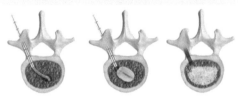

Cavity creation, followed by controlled bone tamp and balloon placement, facilitates central cement filling

| Modular aspects and variations | | |
|---|---|---|
| Curved channel creation | **Curved bone tamp** Balloon variations | |
| Quad-tip needle recovers sample without altering structure | | |
| | Size | 10 | 15 |
| | Maximum inflation volume | 4 mL | 5 mL |
| | Maximum inflated diameter | 16 mm | 16 mm |
| | Maximum inflated length | 20 mm | 28 mm |

| Procedures |
|---|

Kyphoplasty

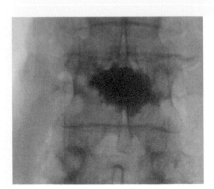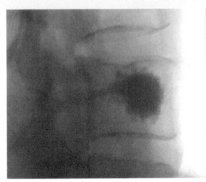

Anteroposterior and lateral fluoroscopic images of Globus Medical AFFIRM® Curved cement placement

**Table 14.6** Globus Medical SHIELD® Vertebral Compression Fracture System

| Design |
|---|

| Specifications |
|---|
| Cement directed into central/anterior body and serves as a physical barrier to posterior elements of spine |

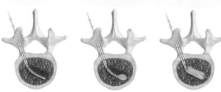

Curved cavity creation prepares pathway across midline of vertebral body into contralateral side

| Modular aspects and variations |
|---|

| Curved channel creation | Shield implant |
|---|---|
| Quad-tip needle recovers sample without altering structure | 15–25 mm (5-mm increments) |

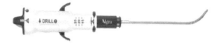 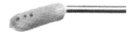

| C3 Curved Cavity Creator functions as a drill and cavity creation instrument | Implant creates an optimized cement column |
|---|---|

| Procedures |
|---|

Vertebroplasty

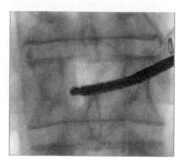 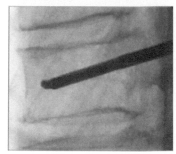

Anteroposterior and lateral fluoroscopic images of Globus Medical SHIELD® C3 Cavity Creator upon insertion

# References

[1] Wang H, Sribastav SS, Ye F, et al. Comparison of percutaneous vertebroplasty and balloon kyphoplasty for the treatment of single level vertebral compression fractures: a meta-analysis of the literature. Pain Physician. 2015; 18(3):209–222

[2] Huang Z, Wan S, Ning L, Han S. Is unilateral kyphoplasty as effective and safe as bilateral kyphoplasties for osteoporotic vertebral compression fractures? A meta-analysis. Clin Orthop Relat Res. 2014; 472(9):2833–2842

[3] Johnell O, Kanis JA. An estimate of the worldwide prevalence and disability associated with osteoporotic fractures. Osteoporos Int. 2006; 17(12):1726–1733

[4] Schlaich C, Minne HW, Bruckner T, et al. Reduced pulmonary function in patients with spinal osteoporotic fractures. Osteoporos Int. 1998; 8(3):261–267

[5] Ensrud KE, Thompson DE, Cauley JA, et al. Fracture Intervention Trial Research Group. Prevalent vertebral deformities predict mortality and hospitalization in older women with low bone mass. J Am Geriatr Soc. 2000; 48(3):241–249

[6] Truumees E, Hilibrand A, VamLaro AR. Percutaneous vertebral augmentation. Spine J. 2004; 4(2):218–229

[7] Yimin Y, Zhiwei R, Wei M, Jha R. Current status of percutaneous vertebroplasty and percutaneous kyphoplasty: a review. Med Sci Monit. 2013; 19:826–836

[8] Shen GW, Wu NQ, Zhang N, Jin ZS, Xu J, Yin GY. A prospective comparative study of kyphoplasty using the Jack vertebral dilator and balloon kyphoplasty for the treatment of osteoporotic vertebral compression fractures. J Bone Joint Surg Br. 2010; 92(9):1282–1288

[9] Deb S. A review of improvements in acrylic bone cements. J Biomater Appl. 1999; 14(1):16–47

[10] Yuan WH, Hsu HC, Lai KL. Vertebroplasty and balloon kyphoplasty versus conservative treatment for osteoporotic vertebral compression fractures: a meta-analysis. Medicine (Baltimore). 2016; 95(31):e4491

[11] Farrokhi MR, Alibai E, Maghami Z. Randomized controlled trial of percutaneous vertebroplasty versus optimal medical management for the relief of pain and disability in acute osteoporotic vertebral compression fractures. J Neurosurg Spine. 2011; 14(5):561–569

[12] Klazen CA, Lohle PN, de Vries J, et al. Vertebroplasty versus conservative treatment in acute osteoporotic vertebral compression fractures (Vertos II): an open-label randomised trial. Lancet. 2010; 376(9746):1085–1092

[13] Zhao S, Xu CY, Zhu AR, et al. Comparison of the efficacy and safety of 3 treatments for patients with osteoporotic vertebral compression fractures: a network meta-analysis. Medicine (Baltimore). 2017; 96(26):e7328

[14] Yaltirik K, Ashour AM, Reis CR, Özdoğan S, Atalay B. Vertebral augmentation by kyphoplasty and vertebroplasty: 8 years experience outcomes and complications. J Craniovertebr Junction Spine. 2016; 7(3):153–160

[15] Tomé-Bermejo F, Piñera AR, Duran-Álvarez C, et al. Identification of risk factors for the omLurrence of cement leakage during percutaneous vertebroplasty for painful osteoporotic or malignant vertebral fracture. Spine. 2014; 39(11):E693–E700

[16] Lin D, Hao J, Li L, et al. Effect of bone cement volume fraction on adjacent vertebral fractures after unilateral percutaneous kyphoplasty. Clin Spine Surg. 2017; 30(3):E270–E275

[17] Chen C, Li D, Wang Z, Li T, Liu X, Zhong J. Safety and efficacy studies of vertebroplasty, kyphoplasty, and mesh-container-plasty for the treatment of vertebral compression fractures: preliminary report. PLoS One. 2016; 11(3):e0151492

[18] Chang X, Lv YF, Chen B, et al. Vertebroplasty versus kyphoplasty in osteoporotic vertebral compression fracture: a meta-analysis of prospective comparative studies. Int Orthop. 2015; 39(3):491–500

[19] Hulme PA, Krebs J, Ferguson SJ, Berlemann U. Vertebroplasty and kyphoplasty: a systematic review of 69 clinical studies. Spine. 2006; 31(17):1983–2001

[20] Heini PF, Wälchli B, Berlemann U. Percutaneous transpedicular vertebroplasty with PMMA: operative technique and early results. A prospective study for the treatment of osteoporotic compression fractures. Eur Spine J. 2000; 9(5):445–450

[21] Santiago FR, Abela AP, Alvarez LG, Osuna RM, García MdelM. Pain and functional outcome after vertebroplasty and kyphoplasty. A comparative study. Eur J Radiol. 2010; 75(2):e108–e113

[22] Ma XL, Xing D, Ma JX, Xu WG, Wang J, Chen Y. Balloon kyphoplasty versus percutaneous vertebroplasty in treating osteoporotic vertebral compression fracture: grading the evidence through a systematic review and meta-analysis. Eur Spine J. 2012; 21(9):1844–1859

[23] Frankel BM, Monroe T, Wang C. Percutaneous vertebral augmentation: an elevation in adjacent-level fracture risk in kyphoplasty as compared with vertebroplasty. Spine J. 2007; 7(5):575–582

[24] Xing D, Ma JX, Ma XL, et al. A meta-analysis of balloon kyphoplasty compared to percutaneous vertebroplasty for treating osteoporotic vertebral compression fractures. J Clin Neurosci. 2013; 20(6):795–803

[25] Yan L, Jiang R, He B, Liu T, Hao D. A comparison between unilateral transverse process-pedicle and bilateral puncture techniques in percutaneous kyphoplasty. Spine. 2014; 39(26 Spec No.):B19–B26

[26] Yan L, He B, Guo H, Liu T, Hao D. The prospective self-controlled study of unilateral transverse process-pedicle and bilateral puncture techniques in percutaneous kyphoplasty. Osteoporos Int. 2016; 27(5):1849–1855

[27] Rebolledo BJ, Gladnick BP, Unnanuntana A, Nguyen JT, Kepler CK, Lane JM. Comparison of unipedicular and bipedicular balloon kyphoplasty for the treatment of osteoporotic vertebral compression fractures: a prospective randomised study. Bone Joint J. 2013; 95-B(3):401–406

[28] Chen L, Yang H, Tang T. Unilateral versus bilateral balloon kyphoplasty for multilevel osteoporotic vertebral compression fractures: a prospective study. Spine. 2011; 36(7):534–540

# 15 Biologics

*Kaitlyn L. Cardinal, Benjamin Khechen, Brittany E. Haws, Jordan A. Guntin,*
*Sravisht Iyer, and Kern Singh*

## 15.1 Introduction

Achieving a solid fusion is crucial to achieving stable, long-term stability following a number of spine surgery procedures.[1,2] Open approaches provide a wide exposure and allow for placement of large quantities of bone graft in the posterolateral gutter. Minimally invasive surgery (MIS) approaches, however, typically require interbody fusion and MIS surgeons frequently use spinal biologics to help achieve this goal.[3] Spinal biologics enhance bone formation via osteoinductive, osteoconductive, osteogenic, or a combination of the three mechanisms.[4,5,6] Osteoinductive biologics stimulate pluripotent stem cells to differentiate into an osteoblastic, bone-forming phenotype. Osteoconductive materials, by contrast, provide a scaffold that supports the growth of new bone. Osteogenesis refers to continued production of bone by preexisting bone-forming cells.

### 15.1.1 Biologics Classification

In most MIS applications, spinal biologics are used in conjunction with an interbody biomechanical device and placed directly in the disk space. The disk space is approached via an anterior, lateral, or posterior approach and prepared for fusion. The interbody device is then loaded with the biologic material and positioned into the disk space to help achieve fusion. There are several choices for the biologically active material that may be placed into the disk space. These can be broadly divided into two categories: bone graft (autograft and allograft) and bone graft extenders (demineralized bone matrix [DBM], bone ceramics, mesenchymal stem cells, and recombinant human bone morphogenetic protein [rhBMP]).

Historically, autograft bone has represented the "gold standard" against which other biologic agents are measured.[3,6,7] Autograft bone may consist of cancellous or corticocancellous bone. In MIS applications, autograft may be obtained from one of the following three sources: iliac crest,[8] bone shavings from an oscillating burr,[9,10] and local bone (laminectomy/facetectomy bone). Autograft bone is considered desirable because it is the only graft choice that is widely accepted to be osteoinductive, osteoconductive, and osteogenic. Allograft bone, in contrast, is osteoconductive and may have some weak osteoinductive effects.[6] For this reason, allograft bone is typically used in conjunction with autograft bone or other osteoinductive agents (e.g., rhBMP). The benefits of allograft bone include the ability to place a larger quantity of bone graft and avoiding any potential donor site morbidity associated with iliac crest bone graft.[11,12] Corticocancellous allograft provides mechanical support in addition to osteoconduction. For this reason, corticocancellous allograft may be placed directly into the interbody space without a cage. This type of allograft is most commonly used in the cervical spine.[13,14]

Bone graft extenders vary in their mechanism of action and efficacy. Major categories of bone graft extenders include DBM, bone ceramics, and rhBMP. DBM is created following chemical extraction of the mineralized portion of cadaveric human bone.[6] This process retains an osteoconductive scaffold for bone growth and also preserves bone proteins such as BMP to provide an osteoinductive effect. Bone ceramics are calcium-based substitutes that provide an osteoconductive scaffold for bone growth.[6,15,16] These graft materials are typically a mix of hydroxyapatite (HA) and tricalcium phosphate (TCP) that undergo gradual remodeling during bone formation.[17]

rhBMP is a widely used adjunct to assist with spinal fusion.[7] BMPs are proteins within the transforming growth factor-beta (TGF-β) superfamily and induce bone formation by inducing the differentiation of pluripotent mesenchymal stem cells toward osteogenic and chondrogenic phenotypes and by stimulating angiogenesis and alkaline phosphatase activity.[17] RhBMP is widely utilized in MIS surgeries via the anterior, lateral, or posterior approaches to assist with interbody fusion.[3,18]

## 15.1.2 Outcomes

Although several authors have examined the use of biologics in open spine surgery, there is less evidence of its use in MIS. The use of autograft in MIS varies by approach, but it is commonly collected and utilized in posterior MIS approaches to the lumbar spine and anterior approaches to the cervical spine. Kasliwal and Deutsch described their results in a series of 40 patients undergoing MIS transforaminal lumbar interbody fusion (TLIF) using a cage filled with local bone shavings.[9] The authors reported a fusion rate of 70% with good clinical outcomes in 92% of patients undergoing a MIS TLIF at minimum 1-year follow-up.[9] In a recently published meta-analysis, Parajón et al reported a 91.8% fusion rate for patients undergoing MIS TLIF with autograft bone only.[3] In these studies, autograft bone typically refers to locally harvested bone (e.g., bone shavings or osteotome cuts). Lopez et al, however, recently described a MIS approach to harvest iliac crest bone.[8] While the early results with this technique are promising, long-term fusion data have not yet been reported.

The use of allograft bone and bone graft extenders is also quite common in the MIS approach. In their meta-analysis, Parajón et al reviewed results from 40 series that spanned 1,533 patients seeking to determine the optimal graft material for MIS TLIF.[3] The authors demonstrated that MIS TLIF resulted in high fusion rates regardless of graft material (91.8–99%), but that the fusion rates generally increased when rhBMP was utilized (96.6 vs. 92.5%). The lowest fusion rates were observed when autologous local bone was utilized without rhBMP or bone graft extenders (91.8%). The addition of rhBMP to local bone increased the fusion rate to 93.1%. Using autograft bone, rhBMP and an additional bone graft extender resulted in fusion rates of 99.1%. It should be noted, however, that this meta-analysis was limited by the substantial heterogeneity in surgical technique, follow-up, and assessment of fusion.[3] Finally, these authors were also unable to determine the clinical significance of fusion in patients undergoing MIS TLIF.[3]

The use of biologic agents is more well established in the anterior lumbar spine, as this was the original indication for which rhBMP was approved.[7] It is generally accepted that in the anterior lumbar spine, the use of rhBMP can result in fusion rates that are noninferior (and potentially superior) to autograft bone.[19,20] Galimberti et al reviewed 16 studies with an rhBMP and control arm to determine the impact of rhBMP on fusion rates in the lumbar spine. The authors stratified their results by approach (anterior lumbar interbody fusion [ALIF], posterior lumbar interbody fusion [PLIF]/TLIF, and posterolateral fusion [PLF]). For ALIF, the authors reported an increase in the rate of fusion in three of four studies (odds ratio: 7.08, 95% confidence interval: 1.5–32.7).[20] The authors determined that there was no increased rate of fusion associated with rhBMP use and PLIF/TLIF.

## 15.1.3 Complications

The use of rhBMP may be associated with several important and clinically relevant complications, including prevertebral swelling in the cervical spine, soft-tissue swelling, local inflammation, cyst formation, osteolysis, implant migration/subsidence, retrograde ejaculation, and ectopic bone formation.[21,22,23,24,25,26,27,28] Ectopic bone formation is an important consideration with the use of BMP in PLIF and TLIF procedures.[29] Although this bone formation is asymptomatic in a majority of cases,[29] it can lead to neuroforaminal impingement and symptoms severe enough to require reoperation.[28]

Singh et al reviewed 610 consecutive patients undergoing an MIS TLIF with BMP and identified a 1.7% rate of reoperation (10/610) in this cohort due to BMP-related complications, including neuroforaminal bone growth, vertebral body osteolysis, and cage migration.[28] All 10 of the patients undergoing reoperation had neuroforaminal stenosis and 2 of the same 10 patients had osteolysis and cage migration. Singh et al also performed a systematic review to examine the complication rates of rhBMP and demonstrated that the rates of complications were highly spine site specific (0.6–20.1% in anterior cervical diskectomy and fusion, 3.5–14.6% in posterior cervical, 2.0–7.3% in ALIFs, and 1.5–21.8% in PLIF/TLIF, and 1.4–8.2% in PLFs). In their analysis, the authors identified that the only individual complication that increased with rhBMP use was retrograde ejaculation.[30,31] It is important to note, however, that the dosing of rhBMP varies widely by institution and surgeon and the complications associated with BMP may be dose dependent.[18]

## 15.2 Bone Ceramics

**Table 15.1** Alphatec Spine Bone X Trudable™ Moldable Synthetic Bone Graft

| Graft specifications | |
|---|---|
| **Composition** | **Design** |
| 60% hydroxyapatite and 40% β-tricalcium phosphate | Microporous and biphasic to promote cellular resorption |
| | Available volumes: 1, 2, 5 mL |

Alphatec Bone X Trudable™ Moldable Synthetic Bone Graft preloaded in syringe

**Table 15.2** Alphatec Spine Neocore™ Osteoconductive Matrix

| Strip technology | |
|---|---|
| **Composition**<br>β-Tricalcium phosphate and type-1 collagen | **Design**<br>Radiopaque, biosynthetic scaffold |

**Strip sizes**

5 cc, 25 × 50 × 4 mm
12 cc, 20 × 100 × 6 mm
20 cc, 25 × 100 × 8 mm

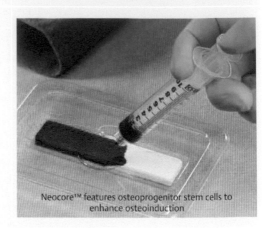

Neocore™ features osteoprogenitor stem cells to enhance osteoinduction

**Table 15.3** Alphatec Spine 3D ProFuse™ Bioscaffold

| Graft technology | |
|---|---|
| **Composition**<br>Demineralized cancellous bone | **Design**<br>Vacuum infusion packaging enables even hydration for homogenous cell distribution |

**Blocks**
9 × 8 × 12 mm
13 × 11 × 11 mm
20 × 6 × 16 mm
22 × 8 × 17 mm
25 × 6 × 16 mm
9 × 9 × 9 mm

**Strips**
25 × 3 × 16 mm
50 × 20 × 3 mm
50 × 20 × 7 mm

**Chips**
1 cc
5 cc
10 cc

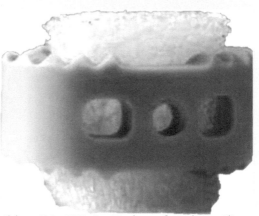

Alphatec Spine 3D ProFuse™ enhances fusion by providing a compressible matrix that facilitates efficient load transfer

**Table 15.4** DePuy Synthes chronOS® Bone Void Filler: Block

| Bone Void Filler specifications | | |
| --- | --- | --- |
| **Composition**<br>β-Tricalcium phosphate | **Porosity**<br>Macropores allow for vascular-<br>ization while micropores<br>increase surface area | **Design**<br>Radiopaque |
| **Available sizes**<br>12.5 × 12.5 × 10 mm<br>20 × 20 × 10 mm | | |

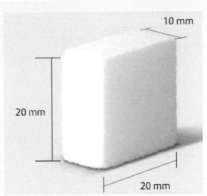

10 mm

20 mm

20 mm

chronOS® Bone Void Filler structure is
designed for bony ingrowth
without loss of stability

**Table 15.5** DePuy Synthes chronOS® Bone Void Filler: Granules

| Bone Void Filler specifications | | |
| --- | --- | --- |
| **Composition**<br>β-Tricalcium phosphate | **Porosity**<br>Macropores allow for vascular-<br>ization, while micropores<br>increase surface area | **Design**<br>Radiopaque |
| **Granule options** | | |

| **Medium**<br>1.4-2.8 mm 5.0, 10.0, 20.0 cc | **Large**<br>2.8-5.6 mm 5.0, 10.0, 20.0 cc |
| --- | --- |

**Table 15.6** DePuy Synthes chronOS® Bone Void Filler: Wedge

| Bone Void Filler specifications | | |
|---|---|---|
| **Composition** | **Porosity** | **Design** |
| β-Tricalcium phosphate | Macropores allow for vascularization while micropores increase surface area | Radiopaque |

| Wedge options | | |
|---|---|---|
| | **Rectangular** | **Semicircular** |
| | | |
| **Length** | 6.5, 8, 10, 12 mm | 7, 10, 13 mm |
| **Width** | 25 mm | 25 mm |
| **Height** | 20 mm | 35 mm |
| **Degree of inclination** | 10, 14, 18, 22° | 7, 10, 13° |

**Table 15.7** K2 M VENADO® Bone Graft System

| Graft technology | |
|---|---|
| **Composition** | **Design** |
| Type I collagen with carbonated calcium phosphate granules | Ceramic and radiopaque |

| Bone graft options | | |
|---|---|---|
| **Blocks** | **Putty** | **Strips** |
| 6.25 × 2 × 0.8 cm | 5-, 10-cc Jar | 12.5 × 2 × 0.4 cm |
| 1 Block: 10 cc | | 1 Strip: 10 cc |
| | | |

Porous structure of K2 M Bone Graft System enhances cellular migration and attachment

**Table 15.8** K2 M VENADO® Foam Strips Bone Graft System

| Graft technology | |
| --- | --- |
| **Composition**<br>60% hydroxyapatite and 40% β-tricalcium phosphate | **Design**<br>Fibrillar collagen and resorbable, radiopaque granules |
| **Available sizes**<br>50 × 10 × 2 mm—1 strip, 1 cc<br>50 × 10 × 5 mm—2 strips, 2 cc<br>50 × 10 × 2 mm—2 strips, 2 cc<br>100 × 25 × 4 mm—1 strip, 10 cc | 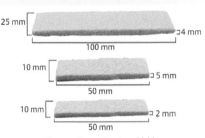<br>Compression resistant, moldable osteoconductive bone scaffold |

**Table 15.9** K2 M VENADO® Granules Bone Graft System

| Graft technology | |
| --- | --- |
| **Composition**<br>60% hydroxyapatite and 40% β-tricalcium phosphate | **Design**<br>Ceramic and radiopaque |
| **Granule sizes**<br><br>0.5–1 mm, 1 cc<br>0.5–1 mm, 2.5 cc<br>1–3 mm, 5 cc<br>1–3 mm, 10 cc<br>1–6 mm, 15 cc<br>1–6 mm, 30 cc | 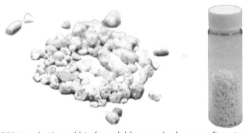 |

100% synthetic and biodegradable granules bone graft system

**Table 15.10** K2 M VESUVIUS® Demineralized Fibers Osteobiologic System

| Graft technology | |
| --- | --- |
| **Allowash XG®** | **PAD®** |
| Sterilization process removes >99% of marrow and blood elements | Demineralization process leaves residual calcium levels of 1–4% |

| Graft specifications | |
| --- | --- |
| **Composition** | |
| Demineralized cortical fibers and mineralized cancellous chips | |
| 100% tissue, contains no fillers | |
| **Fiber sizes** | |
| 2 cc, 5 cc, 15 cc, 30 cc | |

**Table 15.11** K2 M VESUVIUS® Demineralized Sponge Osteobiologic System

| Sponge technology | | |
| --- | --- | --- |
| **Allowash XG®** | | **PAD®** |
| Sterilization process removes > 99% of marrow and blood elements | | Demineralization process leaves residual calcium levels of 1–4% |

| Demineralized sponge options | | |
| --- | --- | --- |
| **Strips** | **Cubes** | **Chips** |
| 10 × 20 × 8 mm | 8 × 8 × 8 mm | 2.5 cc |
| 15 × 20 × 6 mm | 10 × 10 × 10 mm | 5 cc |
| 200 × 25 × 6 mm | 12 × 12 × 12 mm | 10 cc |
| | 14 × 14 × 14 mm | (1–8 mm in size) |

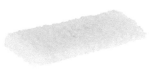  

Cancellous bone tissue available in strip (left), cube (middle), and chip (right) configuration

**Table 15.12** NuVasive Attrax® Putty

| Putty specifications | |
| --- | --- |
| **Composition** | **Design** |
| 90% β-tricalcium phosphate and <10% hydroxyapatite | Biotextured™ surface structure allows for 3D bone regeneration<br>Alkylene oxide copolymer carrier enhances moldability |

Cylinder

8 × 20 mm
1 cc

Cylinder (2)

8 × 20 mm
2 cc

Block (2)

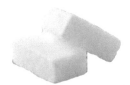

25 × 9 × 13.5 mm
6 cc

Strip (2)

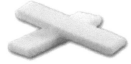

50 × 12.5 × 4 mm
5 cc

Strip (2)

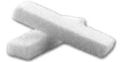

50 × 12.5 × 8 mm
10 cc

**Table 15.13** NuVasive Formagraft® Collagen Bone Graft Matrix

| Graft technology | |
| --- | --- |
| **Composition** | **Design** |
| Purified type 1 collagen and hydroxyapatite, β-tricalcium phosphate granules | Absorbent scaffold enhances cellular migration and controls degradation rate |

| Bone graft options | | |
| --- | --- | --- |
| **Block** | **Strips (2)** | **Granules** |
| Small, large | Small, large | 20 cc |

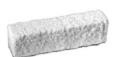

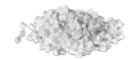

**Table 15.14** NuVasive Osteocel® Pro Allograft Cellular Bone Matrix

| Graft specifications |
| --- |

**Composition**
Demineralized cancellous bone

**Design**
Cohesive and moldable delivery

**Size**
Small, medium, large

**Graft delivery system**
Up to 10 cc of graft delivered per pass

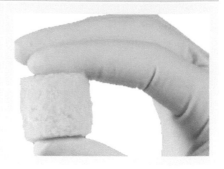

**Table 15.15** SeaSpine Compressible Bone Matrix

| Graft specifications |
| --- |

| **Composition** | **Design** |
| --- | --- |
| Demineralized cancellous bone | Trabecular structure with sponge-like properties promotes compressibility and cellular ingrowth |

**Available sizes**
20 × 15 × 5 mm
20 × 15 × 7 mm
25 × 20 × 7 mm
50 × 20 × 5 mm
10 × 10 × 10 mm
12 × 12 × 12 mm
16 × 16 × 16 mm

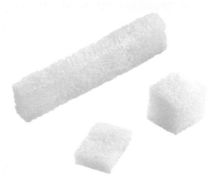

**Table 15.16** Zimmer Biomet CopiOs® Bone Void Filler

| Filler specifications | |
| --- | --- |
| **Composition** | **Design** |
| Calcium phosphate, dibasic, and purified type I bovine collagen | 3D collagen scaffold is 93% porous with interconnecting pores<br>CopiOs® Bone Void Filler promotes moderately acidic environment to stimulate solubility of growth factors |

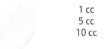

| Filler options | |
| --- | --- |
| **Sponge** | **Paste** |
| 1 × 2 × 0.5 cm, 1 cc<br>2 × 5 × 0.5 cm, 5 cc<br>2 × 5 × 0.2 cm,<br>10 cc (2 units) | 1 cc<br>5 cc<br>10 cc |

**Table 15.17** Zimmer Biomet Indux™ Cancellous Sponge and Cortical Strip

| Cancellous sponge | |
| --- | --- |
| **Composition** | **Design** |
| Demineralized cancellous bone | Trabecular structure allows for cellular infiltration and bone formation |
| **Available sizes**<br>14 × 14 × 14 mm<br>50 × 20 × 5 mm<br>50 × 25 × 8 mm<br>30 × 20 × 5 mm |  |

| Cortical strip | |
| --- | --- |
| **Composition** | **Design** |
| Cortical bone with crosshatch pattern | Channels increase surface area and allow for enhanced vascularization |
| **Available sizes**<br>15 × 11 × 5 mm<br>50 × 14 × 5 mm |  |

**Table 15.18** Zimmer Biomet Pro Osteon® Bone Graft Substitute: Block

| Graft specifications |
| --- |

| Design |
| --- |
| Interconnected porosity for vascular pathways and cell migration |

| 200 and 500 Pro Osteon® Bone Graft Substitute: Block | |
| --- | --- |
| **Composition** | **Porosity** |
| Pure, nonresorbable, hydroxyapatite | 60–70% |

| 200 R and 500 R Pro Osteon® Bone Graft Substitute: Block | |
| --- | --- |
| **Composition** | **Porosity** |
| Hydroxyapatite and calcium carbonate resorb in 6–18 months | 60–70% |

| Pro Osteon® Bone Graft Substitute: Block | | |
| --- | --- | --- |
| **200** | **500** | **500 R** |
| 10 × 10 × 40 mm, 4.0 cc | 40 × 10 × 10 mm, 4.0 cc | 10 × 10 × 10 mm, 1.0 cc |
| 6 × 15 × 50 mm, 4.5 cc | 25 × 25 × 12 mm, 7.5 cc | 40 × 6 × 6 mm, 1.4 cc |
| 10 × 15 × 50 mm, 7.5 cc | 50 × 20 × 10 mm, 10.0 cc | 40 × 12 × 5 mm, 2.4 cc |
| | | 40 × 10 × 10 mm, 4.0 cc |
| | | 25 × 25 × 12 mm, 7.5 cc |
| | | 50 × 20 × 10 mm, 10.0 cc |
| | | 30 × 30 × 12 mm, 10.8 cc |

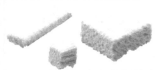

**Table 15.19** Zimmer Biomet Pro Osteon® Bone Graft Substitute: Granules

| Graft specifications |
| --- |

| Design |
| --- |
| Interconnected porosity for vascular pathways and cell migration |

| 200 and 500 Pro Osteon® Bone Graft Substitute: Granules | |
| --- | --- |
| **Composition** | **Porosity** |
| Pure, nonresorbable, hydroxyapatite | 44–45% |

| 200 R and 500 R Pro Osteon® Graft Substitute: Granules | |
| --- | --- |
| **Composition** | **Porosity** |
| Hydroxyapatite and calcium carbonate resorbs in 6–18 months | 60–70% |

| Pro Osteon® Bone Graft Substitute: Granules | | | |
| --- | --- | --- | --- |
| **200** | **200 R** | **500** | **500 R** |
| 2, 5 cc | 0.8, 2, 5, 15 cc | 5, 10, 15, 30 cc | 5, 10, 15, 20, 30 cc |

**Table 15.20** Zimmer Biomet Pro Osteon® Bone Graft Substitute: Wedge

| Graft specifications |
| --- |

| Design |
| --- |
| Interconnected porosity for vascular pathways and cell migration |

| 500 R Pro Osteon® Bone Graft Substitute: Wedge | |
| --- | --- |
| **Composition** | **Porosity** |
| Hydroxyapatite and calcium carbonate resorb in 6–18 months | 60–70% |

| Pro Osteon® Bone Graft Substitute: Wedge | |
| --- | --- |
| **500 R** | |
| Length | 6–20 mm |
| Width | 25 mm |
| Height | 60 mm |
| Degree of Inclination | 3–18° |

**Table 15.21** Zimmer Biomet PlatFORM™ CM Osteoconductive Collagen Mineral Bone Graft Matrix

| Matrix specifications | | | |
|---|---|---|---|
| **Design** Porous structure optimal for interface activity, bone ingrowth, and implant resorption | | | |
| **Matrix options** | | | |
| **Type** | **Putty** | **Block** | **Strip** |
| | Putty | Block | Strip |
| **Composition** | 55% carbonate apatite, 45% collagen | 80% carbonate apatite, 20% collagen | 80% carbonate apatite, 20% collagen |
| **Available Size** | 2 cc 5 cc 10 cc | 6.25 × 2 × 0.4 cm; 5 cc 6.25 × 2 × 0.8 cm; 10 cc 6.25 × 2 × 0.8 cm (2 units); 20 cc | 12.5 × 1 × 0.4 cm; 5 cc 12.5 × 2 × 0.4 cm; 10 cc 12.5 × 2 × 0.4cm (2 units); 20 cc |

# 15.3 Demineralized Bone Matrix

**Table 15.22** Alphatec Spine AlphaGRAFT® C3 Putty

| Putty specifications | |
|---|---|
| **Composition** Demineralized bone with corticocancellous chips and BMP-2 | **Design** Chips provide additional volume and compression resistance |

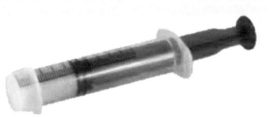

Available volumes: 1.0, 5.0, 10.0 cc

**Table 15.23** Alphatec Spine AlphaGRAFT® DBM

| DBM specifications | |
| --- | --- |
| **Composition** | **Design** |
| Demineralized bone matrix in a biocompatible reverse phase medium | Thickens at body temperature and resists irrigation |

| DBM options | |
| --- | --- |
| Gel | Putty |

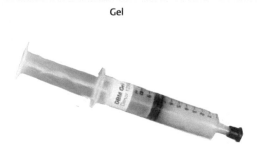

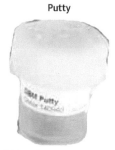

| | |
| --- | --- |
| Available volumes: 1.0, 5.0 cc | Available volumes: 2.5, 5.0, 10.0 cc |

**Table 15.24** DePuy Synthes DBX® Demineralized Bone Matrix: Inject

| Inject features | |
| --- | --- |
| **Composition** | **Design** |
| Granulated cortical bone in sodium hyaluronate | DBX® Demineralized Bone Matrix inject is 31% bone content |

**Available sizes**
2.5 cc
5.0 cc
10.0 cc

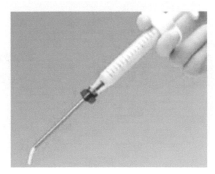

Provides a moldable consistency direct from delivery system

**Table 15.25** DePuy Synthes DBX® Demineralized Bone Matrix: Mix

| Mix features | |
| --- | --- |
| **Composition** | **Design** |
| Demineralized cortical-cancellous bone texture in sodium hyaluronate | Eliminates or reduces need to combine bone chips with DBM<br>DBX® Demineralized Bone Matrix mix is 35% bone content |
| **Available sizes**<br>2.5 cc<br>5.0 cc<br>10.0 cc<br>20.0 cc | 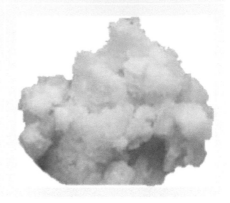 |

**Table 15.26** DePuy Synthes DBX® Demineralized Bone Matrix: Putty

| Putty features | |
| --- | --- |
| **Composition** | **Design** |
| Granulated cortical bone in sodium hyaluronate | DBX® Demineralized Bone Matrix putty is 31% bone content by weight |
| **Available sizes**<br>0.5 cc<br>1.0 cc<br>2.0 cc<br>2.5 cc<br>5.0 cc<br>10.0 cc | 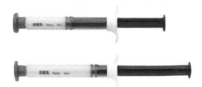<br>Moldable consistency maximizes the amount of bone delivery |

**Table 15.27** DePuy Synthes DBX® Demineralized Bone Matrix: Strip

| Strip features | | |
|---|---|---|
| **Composition** | **Available sizes** | **Design** |
| Demineralized bone, sodium hyaluronate, and gelatin Strip is composed of 45% bone cement | 2.5 × 10 cm 2.5 × 5 cm 5 × 5 cm | Cohesive and flexible consistency to maximize bone delivery to the surgical site |

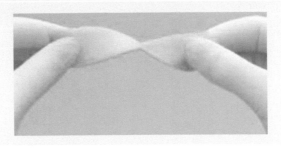

**Table 15.28** DePuy Synthes ViviGen® Cellular Bone Matrix

| Matrix specifications | |
|---|---|
| **Composition** | **Design** |
| Demineralized bone | Corticocancellous chips provide a putty consistency allowing graft to be moldable |
| **ViviGen® volumes** | **ViviGen® formable sizes** |
| 1 cc, 5 cc, 10 cc, 15 cc | Small, medium, large, X-large |

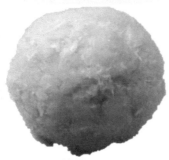

ViviGen

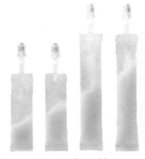

ViviGen formable

**Table 15.29** K2 M VEUVIUS® DBM Putty Osteobiologic System

| Graft technology | |
| --- | --- |
| **Allowash XG®** | **PAD®** |
| Sterilization process removes > 99% of marrow and blood elements | Demineralization process leaves residual calcium levels of 1–4% |

| Graft specifications |
| --- |

**Composition**
Cortical bone-fiber technology combined with glycerol carrier

**Fiber sizes**
1 cc
2.5 cc
5 cc
10 cc

**Table 15.30** K2 M VESUVIUS® DBM Putty 100 Osteobiologic System

| Putty specifications | | |
| --- | --- | --- |
| **Composition** | **Design** | **Available sizes** |
| 100% demineralized allograft tissue | Moldable and irrigation resistant | 0.5, 1, 2.5, 5, 10 cc |

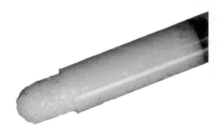

**Table 15.31** NuVasive Propel™ Demineralized Bone Matrix Fibers

| Fiber specifications | |
|---|---|
| **Composition** | **Design** |
| 100% bone | Highly absorbent of physiological fluids |
| | Propel™ demineralized bone matrix fibers offer |
| | continuous 3D architecture for bone formation |
| **Available sizes** | |
| 50 × 25 mm; 5 cc | 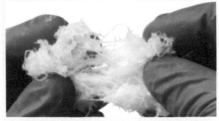 |
| 100 × 25 mm; 20 cc | |

**Table 15.32** NuVasive Propel™ Demineralized Bone Matrix Putty

| Putty specifications | |
|---|---|
| **Composition** | **Design** |
| Demineralized bone matrix in reverse phase medium | Hardens in situ and resists irrigation |

Propel™ demineralized bone matrix is easily moldable and fits securely into voids

**Table 15.33** SeaSpine OsteoSparx® and OsteoSparx® C

| Graft specifications | |
| --- | --- |
| **Composition** | **Design** |
| Demineralized bone matrix with or without cancellous bone | Reverse phase medium enhances malleability at room temperature |

| Graft options | |
| --- | --- |
| Putty | Gel |

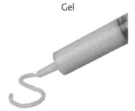

| | |
| --- | --- |
| OsteoSparx® available volumes: 1, 2.5, 5, 10 cc | OsteoSparx® available volumes: 1, 5, 10 cc |
| OsteoSparx® C available volumes: 5, 10 cc | OsteoSparx® C available volumes: 1, 3, 8 cc |

**Table 15.34** SeaSpine Spine Pure Strip Allograft

| Strip specifications | |
| --- | --- |
| **Composition** | **Design** |
| 100% demineralized bone matrix tissue | Pliable and conforms to defect site for enhanced contact with bone |

**Available sizes**
5 cm × 2.5 cm, 6 cc
10 cm × 2.5 cm, 12 cc
10 cm × 1 cm, 16 cc (2 units)

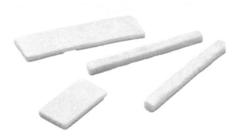

**Table 15.35** SeaSpine OsteoSurge® 100

| Putty specifications | |
|---|---|
| **Composition** | **Design** |
| Demineralized bone matrix incorporated with Accell Bone Matrix | Reverse phase medium enhances malleability at room temperature |

**Available volumes**
1 cc
2.5 cc
5 cc
10 cc

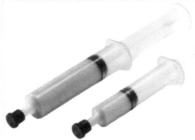

Accell Bone Matrix allows for increased porosity and greater exposure to bone proteins

**Table 15.36** SeaSpine OsteoSurge® 300 and 300 c

| Putty specifications | |
|---|---|
| **Composition** | **Design** |
| Demineralized bone matrix incorporated with Accell Bone Matrix<br>300 c contains cancellous chips to create a porous structure | Reverse phase medium (RPM) enhances malleability<br>Thermoreversibility enhances irrigation resistance |

**Available volumes**
1 cc
2.5 cc
5 cc
10 cc

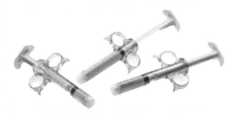

**Table 15.37** Zimmer Biomet InterGro® DBM

| DMB specifications | |
| --- | --- |
| **Composition** | **Design** |
| Demineralized bone matrix in natural lecithin carrier | Natural lipid carrier resistant to breakdown |

| DBM options |
| --- |

**Putty**
40% DBM
Volumes available: 10 cc

**Paste**
35% DBM
Volumes available: 0.5, 1, 2, 5 cc

**Plus**
35% DBM premixed with coralline hydroxyapatite and calcium carbonate
Volumes available: 2, 5, 10 cc

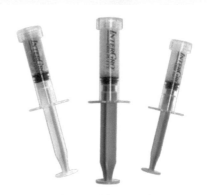

**Table 15.38** Zimmer Biomet Puros® Demineralized Bone Matrix (DBM)

| Block and strip | |
| --- | --- |
| **Composition** | **Design** |
| 100% demineralized cancellous bone | Retains endogenous growth factors BMP-2, BMP-4, and BMP-7 |

Block

12 × 12 × 12mm
14 × 14 × 14mm

Strip

15 × 49 × 3–6mm
20 × 50 × 3–6mm

**Table 15.38** (*Continued*) Zimmer Biomet Puros® Demineralized Bone Matrix (DBM)

| DMB with reverse phase medium (RPM) family products | |
| --- | --- |
| **Composition** <br> Demineralized bone matrix in RPM | **Design** <br> Malleable, viscous at body temperature, resists irrigation |

| Putty | Putty with chips | Gel | Paste |
| --- | --- | --- | --- |
| 1 cc <br> 2.5 cc <br> 5 cc <br> 10 cc | 5 cc <br> 10 cc | 1 cc <br> 5 cc <br> 10 cc | 1 cc <br> 3 cc <br> 8 cc |

# 15.4 Structural Allograft

**Table 15.39** K2 M VIKOS® Shafts Allograft System

| Graft technology | |
| --- | --- |
| **Allowash XG®** <br> Sterilization process removes > 99% of marrow and blood elements | **Preservon®** <br> Ambient temperature storage preservation solution |

| Allograft options | |
| --- | --- |
| **Femoral shaft** <br> For use in lumbar corpectomies <br> Lengths: 60, 100 mm | **Fibular shaft** <br> Processed from the fibula, radius, or ulna <br> Lengths: 20, 40, 60, 100 mm |

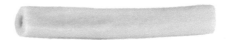

| Femoral shaft | Fibular shaft |
| --- | --- |

**Table 15.40** K2 M VIKOS® Void Fillers Allograft System

| Graft technology | | |
|---|---|---|
| **Allowash XG®** Sterilization process removes >99% of marrow and blood elements | | **Preservon®** Ambient temperature storage preservation solution |
| **Void filler chip options** | | |
| | Course grind | Medium grind |
| Particle size | 1–8 mm | 1–4 mm |
| Bone type | Cancellous and corticocancellous | Cancellous |
| Volumes | 15,* 30, 60 cc (*cancellous only) | 15, 30, 60 cc |

| Coarse cancellous | Coarse corticocancellous | Medium cancellous |

**Table 15.41** SeaSpine Allograft

| Allograft specifications | |
| --- | --- |
| **Composition**<br>Cancellous bone | **Design**<br>Porous scaffold enabling attachment, migration, and distribution of osteogenic and vascular cells |

| Allograft options | |
| --- | --- |
| Crushed | Chips |

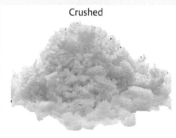

Size ranges: 1–4 mm; 15 cc, 30 cc

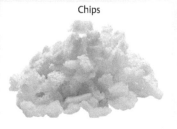

Size ranges: 4–10mm; 15 cc, 30 cc

**Table 15.42** Zimmer Biomet Cellentra® Advanced Allograft

| Graft technology |
| --- |

**Composition**
Cancellous bone and demineralized cortical bone

**Design**
Interconnected trabecular structure
Includes BMP-2, -4, -6, -7, VEGF, TGF-β, PDGF, IGF-1, FG-1, -2

Cellentra® Advanced Allograft features
freshfrozen cryopreserved design

**Table 15.43** Zimmer Biomet PrimaGen Advanced™ Allograft

| Allograft specifications | |
| --- | --- |
| **Composition** | **Design** |
| Demineralized cortical bone fibers and cancellous bone | Interconnected trabecular structure<br>Includes BMP-2, -4, -6, -7, VEGF, TGF-β, PDGF, IGF-1, FG-3, -4 |
| **Available sizes**<br>1 cc<br>5 cc<br>10 cc<br>15 cc | |

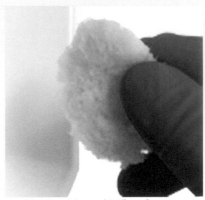

PrimaGen Advanced™ Allograft creates interface activity, bone ingrowth, and graft remodeling

# References

[1] Kornblum MB, Fischgrund JS, Herkowitz HN, Abraham DA, Berkower DL, Ditkoff JS. Degenerative lumbar spondylolisthesis with spinal stenosis: a prospective long-term study comparing fusion and pseudarthrosis. Spine. 2004; 29(7):726–733, discussion 733–734

[2] Fischer CR, Ducoffe AR, Errico TJ. Posterior lumbar fusion: choice of approach and adjunct techniques. J Am Acad Orthop Surg. 2014; 22(8):503–511

[3] Parajón A, Alimi M, Navarro-Ramirez R, et al. Minimally invasive transforaminal lumbar interbody fusion: meta-analysis of the fusion rates. What is the optimal graft material? Neurosurgery. 2017; 81(6):958–971

[4] Grabowski G, Cornett CA. Bone graft and bone graft substitutes in spine surgery: current concepts and controversies. J Am Acad Orthop Surg. 2013; 21(1):51–60

[5] Albrektsson T, Johansson C. Osteoinduction, osteoconduction and osseointegration. Eur Spine J. 2001; 10 Suppl 2:S96–S101

[6] Kannan A, Dodwad S-NM, Hsu WK. Biologics in spine arthrodesis. J Spinal Disord Tech. 2015; 28(5):163–170

[7] Rihn JA, Gates C, Glassman SD, Phillips FM, Schwender JD, Albert TJ. The use of bone morphogenetic protein in lumbar spine surgery. Instr Course Lect. 2009; 58:677–688

[8] Lopez GD, Hijji FY, Narain AS, Yom KH, Singh K. Iliac crest bone graft: a minimally invasive harvesting technique. Clin Spine Surg. 2017; 30(10):439–441

[9] Kasliwal MK, Deutsch H. Clinical and radiographic outcomes using local bone shavings as autograft in minimally invasive transforaminal lumbar interbody fusion. World Neurosurg. 2012; 78(1–2):185–190

[10] Eder C, Chavanne A, Meissner J, et al. Autografts for spinal fusion: osteogenic potential of laminectomy bone chips and bone shavings collected via high speed drill. Eur Spine J. 2011; 20(11):1791–1795

[11] Banwart JC, Asher MA, Hassanein RS. Iliac crest bone graft harvest donor site morbidity. A statistical evaluation. Spine. 1995; 20(9):1055–1060

[12] Summers BN, Eisenstein SM. Donor site pain from the ilium. A complication of lumbar spine fusion. J Bone Joint Surg Br. 1989; 71(4):677–680

[13] An HS, Simpson JM, Glover JM, Stephany J. Comparison between allograft plus demineralized bone matrix versus autograft in anterior cervical fusion. A prospective multicenter study. Spine. 1995; 20(20):2211–2216

[14] Chau AMT, Mobbs RJ. Bone graft substitutes in anterior cervical discectomy and fusion. Eur Spine J. 2009; 18(4):449–464

[15] Zadegan SA, Abedi A, Jazayeri SB, Bonaki HN, Vaccaro AR, Rahimi-Movaghar V. Clinical application of ceramics in anterior cervical discectomy and fusion: a review and update. Global Spine J. 2017; 7(4):343–349

[16] Nickoli MS, Hsu WK. Ceramic-based bone grafts as a bone grafts extender for lumbar spine arthrodesis: a systematic review. Global Spine J. 2014; 4(3):211–216

[17] Campana V, Milano G, Pagano E, et al. Bone substitutes in orthopaedic surgery: from basic science to clinical practice. J Mater Sci Mater Med. 2014; 25(10):2445–2461

[18] Hofstetter CP, Hofer AS, Levi AD. Exploratory meta-analysis on dose-related efficacy and morbidity of bone morphogenetic protein in spinal arthrodesis surgery. J Neurosurg Spine. 2016; 24(3):457–475

[19] Faundez A, Tournier C, Garcia M, Aunoble S, Le Huec J-C. Bone morphogenetic protein use in spine surgery-complications and outcomes: a systematic review. Int Orthop. 2016; 40(6):1309–1319

[20] Galimberti F, Lubelski D, Healy AT, et al. A systematic review of lumbar fusion rates with and without the use of rhBMP-2. Spine. 2015; 40(14):1132–1139

[21] Xu R, Bydon M, Sciubba DM, et al. Safety and efficacy of rhBMP2 in posterior cervical spinal fusion for subaxial degenerative spine disease: analysis of outcomes in 204 patients. Surg Neurol Int. 2011; 2:109

[22] Singh K, Marquez-Lara A, Nandyala SV, Patel AA, Fineberg SJ. Incidence and risk factors for dysphagia after anterior cervical fusion. Spine. 2013; 38(21):1820–1825

[23] Molinari RW, Molinari C. The use of bone morphogenetic protein in pediatric cervical spine fusion surgery: case reports and review of the literature. Global Spine J. 2016; 6(1):e41–e46

[24] Bess S, Line BG, Lafage V, et al. International Spine Study Group ISSG. Does recombinant human bone morphogenetic protein-2 use in adult spinal deformity increase complications and are complications associated with location of rhBMP-2 use? A prospective, multicenter study of 279 consecutive patients. Spine. 2014; 39(3):233–242

[25] Goode AP, Richardson WJ, Schectman RM, Carey TS. Complications, revision fusions, readmissions, and utilization over a 1-year period after bone morphogenetic protein use during primary cervical spine fusions. Spine J. 2014; 14(9):2051–2059

[26] Simmonds MC, Brown JV, Heirs MK, et al. Safety and effectiveness of recombinant human bone morphogenetic protein-2 for spinal fusion: a meta-analysis of individual-participant data. Ann Intern Med. 2013; 158(12):877–889

[27] Cahill KS, Chi JH, Day A, Claus EB. Prevalence, complications, and hospital charges associated with use of bone-morphogenetic proteins in spinal fusion procedures. JAMA. 2009; 302(1):58–66

[28] Singh K, Nandyala SV, Marquez-Lara A, et al. Clinical sequelae after rhBMP-2 use in a minimally invasive transforaminal lumbar interbody fusion. Spine J. 2013; 13(9):1118–1125

[29] Wong DA, Kumar A, Jatana S, Ghiselli G, Wong K. Neurologic impairment from ectopic bone in the lumbar canal: a potential complication of off-label PLIF/TLIF use of bone morphogenetic protein-2 (BMP-2). Spine J. 2008; 8(6):1011–1018

[30] Singh K, Ahmadinia K, Park DK, et al. Complications of spinal fusion with utilization of bone morphogenetic protein: a systematic review of the literature. Spine. 2014; 39(1):91–101

[31] Carragee EJ, Mitsunaga KA, Hurwitz EL, Scuderi GJ. Retrograde ejaculation after anterior lumbar interbody fusion using rhBMP-2: a cohort controlled study. Spine J. 2011; 11(6):511–516

# 16 Surgical Navigation Systems

*Simon P. Lalehzarian, Benjamin Khechen, Brittany E. Haws, Kaitlyn L. Cardinal, Jordan A. Guntin, and Kern Singh*

## 16.1 Introduction

Intraoperative imaging used in the placement of posterior pedicle screws is especially crucial in minimally invasive surgery where direct visualization of anatomic structures is limited. The conventional technique used by the majority of surgeons is fluoroscopy, which involves the introduction of a C-arm into the surgical field. However, conventional fluoroscopic imaging has been associated with variable screw placement accuracy and concerns regarding radiation exposure for the patient and operative staff.[1,2,3,4,5,6] Inaccurate screw placement can lead to severe neurovascular injury with significant perioperative morbidity. Excessive radiation exposure has also been associated with increased risks of teratogenesis and carcinogenesis.[7,8,9,10,11] As a result, image-guided navigation systems have been developed with the goals of improving screw placement accuracy and reducing operative radiation exposure.

Spinal navigation provides real-time, image-based guidance for insertion of pedicle screws and other spinal instrumentation. In this process, radiographic images of the anatomy of interest are uploaded into a computer workstation to produce a three-dimensional (3D) reconstruction of the relevant anatomy that can be viewed preoperatively or intraoperatively. This real-time display of the anatomy is also supplemented with specialized surgical tools whose positions and trajectories can be detected by the system and displayed to the surgeon.[12] This real-time visualization of surgical anatomy and tools allows for insertion of instrumentation without the need to acquire multiple fluoroscopic images.

## 16.2 Components

### 16.2.1 Imaging Modalities

Navigation systems utilize multiple imaging modalities to acquire the necessary anatomical images. Fluoroscopy-based techniques can be adapted, using either two-dimensional (2D) or 3D modalities. Computed tomography (CT)-based techniques include 2D intraoperative CT (iCT), cone-beam 3D CT with a 190° scanning arc, or O-arm imaging with a 360° scanning arc. Additional techniques also include intraoperative magnetic resonance imaging (MRI) or ultrasonography. Imaging can be performed either preoperatively or intraoperatively, with subsequent uploading of the data into the navigation workstation.

### 16.2.2 Workstation

The navigation workstation contains multiple components essential for successful implementation of image guidance. The workstation houses a computer system containing software that integrates radiographic imaging studies, produces 3D anatomic reconstructions, and allows for positional tracking of specialized surgical instruments. The workstation also contains a camera, which is utilized to detect the position of reference frames and surgical instruments within the operative field. This camera can use a variety of different detection modalities, including optical imaging, electromagnetic detection, or acoustic detection.[13] Workstations also contain high-resolution display screens which can be viewed from the operating table, allowing the surgical staff to analyze the patient's anatomy and the instrument positions to determine the optimal trajectories for insertion of instrumentation.

## 16.2.3 Dynamic Reference Frames

Dynamic reference frames interact with the workstation's camera and aid in positional tracking. These constructs are affixed onto anatomical landmarks within the surgical field, and act as a point of reference for the workstation's camera system to determine the position of navigated instruments in relation to the patient's anatomy. Most commonly, these reference frames are directly affixed to bony landmarks within the surgical field such as the spinous processes or the posterior superior iliac spine.[14]

## 16.2.4 Surgical Navigation Instruments

Navigation systems use specialized surgical instruments that are outfitted with tracking sensors or transmitters that are detected by the workstation's camera.[15] The navigation system then uses this information to plot the position and trajectory of these instruments in relation to dynamic reference frames and the patient's anatomy. Instrument position is displayed in real time on the navigation screen, superimposed on the imaging studies or 3D anatomic reconstructions produced by the workstation. This capability allows for updatable, real-time guidance of instrument position to determine the optimal trajectory for insertion of spinal instrumentation.

# 16.3 Outcomes

The clinical efficacy of navigation systems is primarily measured against and compared to pedicle screw insertion accuracy rates seen in procedures done with conventional fluoroscopy. Multiple large meta-analyses have been performed that have demonstrated higher pedicle screw insertion accuracy in cases using spinal navigation.[1,2,16,17] Mason et al, in a meta-analysis of 30 studies comparing conventional fluoroscopy to both 2D and 3D fluoroscopy-guided navigation, found significant differences in accuracy among the modalities.[1] Navigation using either modality had a statistically higher rate of screw accuracy compared to conventional fluoroscopy, and this pattern was seen at all thoracic and lumbosacral spinal levels tested. Shin et al noted similar findings pertaining to accuracy, with navigated operations having an accuracy of 93.3% compared to 84.7% in nonnavigated procedures ($p < 0.001$).[17] Furthermore, no neurologic complications were described in 719 navigation patients, while 2.3% of patients undergoing a procedure with conventional fluoroscopy experienced postoperative neurologic deficits. Shin et al further demonstrated the improved accuracy and complication profile of navigated procedures, while also determining that navigated and nonnavigated procedures had no statistical differences in operative time and intraoperative blood loss.

Spinal navigation systems demonstrate the advantage of intraoperative radiation exposure reduction. One manner by which navigation systems possibly reduce radiation dosage is by allowing surgical team members to exit the operating room during image acquisition and registration.[18] This is especially true when preoperative images are used, or when CT-guided intraoperative imaging systems such as isocentric 3D C-arms and O-arms are used. Regarding measured intraoperative exposure, multiple studies have demonstrated significant, quantifiable reductions in radiation exposure to the surgeon and operative room staff when navigation is used compared to nonnavigated procedures.[10,18,19,20,21,22,23,24,25]

Trends in the usage of navigation have also led to the increasing utilization of intraoperative 3D imaging modalities over preoperative imaging studies. This trend has occurred because of the distinct advantages offered by intraoperative imaging techniques. Intraoperative imaging also provides a better representation of surgical anatomy compared to preoperative imaging, which is typically not acquired in surgical positions and is subject to anatomical shifts.[26,27,28,29,30] Furthermore, intraoperative imaging can be repeated as necessary, allowing for updates that take into account the positional shifts and anatomical manipulations that occur during procedures.[31] The advent of automated registration of images within the workstation eliminates the necessity for the time-consuming point or surface matching required during registration of preoperative images.[31,32,33,34,35] In a study investigating the accuracy of pedicle screw placement in the cervicothoracic spine, Scheufler et al demonstrated that iCT-based spinal navigation with automated registration allowed for safe multisegmental instrumentation of up to 10 contiguous segments.[36] Additionally, the authors demonstrated the use of iCT significantly reduced the need for reregistration in multilevel surgery.

**Table 16.1** Medtronic StealthStation™ S8 Surgical Navigation System

| System overview | |
| --- | --- |
| **Software/Devices** | **Imaging modalities** |
| Utilizes a combination of hardware, software, tracking algorithms, image data merging, and specialized instruments with Dual Cart Stealth S8 System and O-arm Surgical Imaging System | Preoperative planning and intraoperative navigation with iMRI, iCT; can wirelessly import to hospital and medical devices |

| System features |
| --- |
| The Dual Cart Stealth S8 System has two monitors that provide ultimate flexibility and allows for large tracking volume of surgical instrumentation via optical or electromagnetic navigation options |
| O-arm Surgical Imaging System provides intraoperative 3D navigation for confirmation of implant placement and automatic patient registration before leaving operating room |

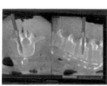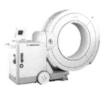

Medtronic StealthStation™ S8 Surgical Navigation System with software display, and O-arm Surgical Imaging Unit (right)

| Procedures |
| --- |
| MIS TLIF, MIS LLIF, MIS posterior decompression |

# 16.4 Surgical Navigation Systems

**Table 16.2** NuVasive Integrated Global Alignment (iGA)

| System overview | |
|---|---|
| **Software/Devices** | **Imaging modalities** |
| Utilizes NuvaPlanning technology (NuvaLine, NuvaMap, and NuvaMap O.R.) and NuVasive NVM5® Platform | Preoperative: CT images with parameter measurements are imported to NVM5® Platform via USB from NuvaMap or manually from NuvaLine Intraoperative: fluoroscopic images from a compatible C-arm imaging unit are imported to NVM5® Platform |

**System features**

NuvaLine allows for preoperative parameter measurements on iPhone/iPad using CT images
NuvaMap simulates surgical options and allows for preoperative parameter measurements with mobile or desktop versions using CT images
NuvaMap O.R. allows for real-time intraoperative assessment of alignment values using fluoroscopic images

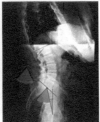 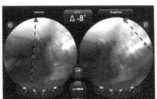

NuVasive NuvaLine (left) and NuVasive NuvaMap (right)

**Procedures**

MIS TLIF, MIS LLIF, MIS posterior decompression

**Table 16.3** Ziehm Imaging Vision RFD 3D

| System overview | |
| --- | --- |
| **Software/Devices** | **Imaging modalities** |
| Utilizes Stryker NAV3i Surgical Navigation Platform, Ziehm Vision RFD 3D C-arm, and Ziehm NaviPort Interface | Intraoperative: Ziehm Vision RFD 3D offers 2D and 3D imaging that delivers CT-like reconstructions to the Stryker NAV3i Surgical Navigation Platform via the Ziehm NaviPort Interface |

| System features |
| --- |
| Stryker NAV3i Surgical Navigation Platform tracks position of the patient and the Ziehm Vision RFD 3D C-arm |
| Ziehm Vision RFD 3D is a mobile and highly flexible C-arm that is significantly smaller than fixed C-arms and is 60% lighter than mobile CTs allowing for simplified positioning in the operating room |

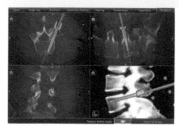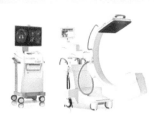

Stryker NAV3i Surgical Navigation Platform display (left) and Ziehm Vision RFD 3D C-arm imaging unit (right)

| Procedures |
| --- |
| MIS TLIF, MIS LLIF, MIS posterior decompression |

# References

[1] Mason A, Paulsen R, Babuska JM, et al. The accuracy of pedicle screw placement using intraoperative image guidance systems. J Neurosurg Spine. 2014; 20(2):196–203

[2] Moses ZB, Mayer RR, Strickland BA, et al. Neuronavigation in minimally invasive spine surgery. Neurosurg Focus. 2013; 35(2):E12

[3] Rampersaud YR, Foley KT, Shen AC, Williams S, Solomito M. Radiation exposure to the spine surgeon during fluoroscopically assisted pedicle screw insertion. Spine. 2000; 25(20):2637–2645

[4] Singer G. Occupational radiation exposure to the surgeon. J Am Acad Orthop Surg. 2005; 13(1):69–76

[5] Theocharopoulos N, Perisinakis K, Damilakis J, Papadokostakis G, Hadjipavlou A, Gourtsoyiannis N. Occupational exposure from common fluoroscopic projections used in orthopaedic surgery. J Bone Joint Surg Am. 2003; 85(9):1698–1703

[6] Ul Haque M, Shufflebarger HL, O'Brien M, Macagno A. Radiation exposure during pedicle screw placement in adolescent idiopathic scoliosis: Is fluoroscopy safe? Spine. 2006; 31(21):2516–2520

[7] Dewey P, Incoll I. Evaluation of thyroid shields for reduction of radiation exposure to orthopaedic surgeons. Aust N Z J Surg. 1998; 68(9):635–636

[8] Giordano BD, Baumhauer JF, Morgan TL, Rechtine GR, II. Cervical spine imaging using mini–C-arm fluoroscopy: patient and surgeon exposure to direct and scatter radiation. J Spinal Disord Tech. 2009; 22(6):399–403

[9] Mastrangelo G, Fedeli U, Fadda E, Giovanazzi A, Scoizzato L, Saia B. Increased cancer risk among surgeons in an orthopaedic hospital. Occup Med (Lond). 2005; 55(6):498–500

[10] Mendelsohn D, Strelzow J, Dea N, et al. Patient and surgeon radiation exposure during spinal instrumentation using intraoperative computed tomography-based navigation. Spine J. 2016; 16(3):343–354

[11] Perisinakis K, Theocharopoulos N, Damilakis J, et al. Estimation of patient dose and associated radiogenic risks from fluoroscopically guided pedicle screw insertion. Spine. 2004; 29(14):1555–1560

[12] Nolte LP, Visarius H, Arm E, Langlotz F, Schwarzenbach O, Zamorano L. Computer-aided fixation of spinal implants. J Image Guid Surg. 1995; 1(2):88–93

[13] Manbachi A, Cobbold RS, Ginsberg HJ. Guided pedicle screw insertion: techniques and training. Spine J. 2014; 14(1):165–179

[14] Cho JY, Chan CK, Lee SH, Lee HY. The accuracy of 3D image navigation with a cutaneously fixed dynamic reference frame in minimally invasive transforaminal lumbar interbody fusion. Comput Aided Surg. 2012; 17(6):300–309

[15] Cleary K, Peters TM. Image-guided interventions: technology review and clinical applications. Annu Rev Biomed Eng. 2010; 12:119–142

[16] Verma R, Krishan S, Haendlmayer K, Mohsen A. Functional outcome of computer-assisted spinal pedicle screw placement: a systematic review and meta-analysis of 23 studies including 5,992 pedicle screws. Eur Spine J. 2010; 19(3):370–375

[17] Shin BJ, James AR, Njoku IU, Härtl R. Pedicle screw navigation: a systematic review and meta-analysis of perforation risk for computer-navigated versus freehand insertion. J Neurosurg Spine. 2012; 17(2):113–122

[18] Kim CW, Lee YP, Taylor W, Oygar A, Kim WK. Use of navigation-assisted fluoroscopy to decrease radiation exposure during minimally invasive spine surgery. Spine J. 2008; 8(4):584–590

[19] Bandela JR, Jacob RP, Arreola M, Griglock TM, Bova F, Yang M. Use of CT-based intraoperative spinal navigation: management of radiation exposure to operator, staff, and patients. World Neurosurg. 2013; 79(2):390–394

[20] Hott JS, Papadopoulos SM, Theodore N, Dickman CA, Sonntag VK. Intraoperative Iso-C C-arm navigation in cervical spinal surgery: review of the first 52 cases. Spine. 2004; 29(24):2856–2860

[21] Lange J, Karellas A, Street J, et al. Estimating the effective radiation dose imparted to patients by intraoperative cone-beam computed tomography in thoracolumbar spinal surgery. Spine. 2013; 38(5):E306–E312

[22] Nottmeier EW, Pirris SM, Edwards S, Kimes S, Bowman C, Nelson KL. Operating room radiation exposure in cone beam computed tomography-based, image-guided spinal surgery: clinical article. J Neurosurg Spine. 2013; 19(2):226–231

[23] Pitteloud N, Gamulin A, Barea C, Damet J, Racloz G, Sans-Merce M. Radiation exposure using the O-arm(R) surgical imaging system. Eur Spine J. 2017; 26(3):651–657

[24] Smith HE, Welsch MD, Sasso RC, Vaccaro AR. Comparison of radiation exposure in lumbar pedicle screw placement with fluoroscopy vs computer-assisted image guidance with intraoperative three-dimensional imaging. J Spinal Cord Med. 2008; 31(5):532–537

[25] Tabaraee E, Gibson AG, Karahalios DG, Potts EA, Mobasser JP, Burch S. Intraoperative cone beam-computed tomography with navigation (O-ARM) versus conventional fluoroscopy (C-arm): a cadaveric study comparing accuracy, efficiency, and safety for spinal instrumentation. Spine. 2013; 38(22):1953–1958

[26] Beck M, Mittlmeier T, Gierer P, Harms C, Gradl G. Benefit and accuracy of intraoperative 3D-imaging after pedicle screw placement: a prospective study in stabilizing thoracolumbar fractures. Eur Spine J. 2009; 18(10):1469–1477

[27] Ebmeier K, Giest K, Kalff R. Intraoperative computerized tomography for improved accuracy of spinal navigation in pedicle screw placement of the thoracic spine. Acta Neurochir Suppl (Wien). 2003; 85:105–113

[28] Holly LT, Foley KT. Three-dimensional fluoroscopy-guided percutaneous thoracolumbar pedicle screw placement. Technical note. J Neurosurg. 2003; 99(3) Suppl:324–329

[29] Nakashima H, Sato K, Ando T, Inoh H, Nakamura H. Comparison of the percutaneous screw placement precision of isocentric C-arm 3-dimensional fluoroscopy-navigated pedicle screw implantation and conventional fluoroscopy method with minimally invasive surgery. J Spinal Disord Tech. 2009; 22(7):468–472

[30] Nottmeier EW, Seemer W, Young PM. Placement of thoracolumbar pedicle screws using three-dimensional image guidance: experience in a large patient cohort. J Neurosurg Spine. 2009; 10(1):33–39

[31] Gebhard F, Weidner A, Liener UC, Stöckle U, Arand M. Navigation at the spine. Injury. 2004; 35 Suppl 1: S-A35–S-A45

[32] Scheufler KM, Cyron D, Dohmen H, Eckardt A. Less invasive surgical correction of adult degenerative scoliosis, part I: technique and radiographic results. Neurosurgery. 2010; 67(3):696–710

[33] Tormenti MJ, Kostov DB, Gardner PA, Kanter AS, Spiro RM, Okonkwo DO. Intraoperative computed tomography image-guided navigation for posterior thoracolumbar spinal instrumentation in spinal deformity surgery. Neurosurg Focus. 2010; 28(3):E11

[34] Uhl E, Zausinger S, Morhard D, et al. Intraoperative computed tomography with integrated navigation system in a multidisciplinary operating suite. Neurosurgery. 2009; 64(5) Suppl 2:231–239, discussion 239–240

[35] Zausinger S, Scheder B, Uhl E, Heigl T, Morhard D, Tonn JC. Intraoperative computed tomography with integrated navigation system in spinal stabilizations. Spine. 2009; 34(26):2919–2926

[36] Scheufler KM, Franke J, Eckardt A, Dohmen H. Accuracy of image-guided pedicle screw placement using intraoperative computed tomography-based navigation with automated referencing, part I: cervicothoracic spine. Neurosurgery. 2011; 69(4):782–795, discussion 795

# Index

## A

abdominal musculature, 121
Alphatec Spine 3D ProFuse™ Bioscaffold, 194
Alphatec Spine AlphaGRAFT® C3 Putty, 204
Alphatec Spine AlphaGRAFT® DBM, 205
Alphatec Spine Arsenal™ CBx Cortical Bone Fixation System, 90
Alphatec Spine Battalion™ PC, 57
Alphatec Spine Battalion™ PS, 58
Alphatec Spine Bone X Trudable™ Moldable Synthetic Bone Graft, 193
Alphatec Spine BridgePoint® Spinous Process Fixation System, 107
Alphatec Spine Illico® FS Facet Fixation System, 98
Alphatec Spine Illico® MIS Posterior Fixation System, 76
Alphatec Spine Illico® Posterior Thoracolumbar Retractor System, 17
Alphatec Spine Neocore™ Osteoconductive Matrix, 194
Alphatec Spine Novel® CP Spinal Spacer System, 160
Alphatec Spine Novel® SD, 29, 48
Alphatec Spine Novel® Tapered TL, 30
Autograft bone, 191

## B

balloon kyphoplasty, 181
Benvenue Medical Kiva® Vertebral Compression Fracture Treatment System, 183
Benvenue Medical Luna™ 3D, 66
Biologics
– bone ceramics, 193–216
– classification, 191–192
– complications, 193
– outcomes, 192
Bipolar cautery, 122
Bladed retractors, 11
bone ceramics, 193–216
Bone graft extenders, 191
bone graft extenders, 192
Bone grafts, 156

## C

Cannulated screws, 74
cannulated trocar, 180
carbon fiber, 157
cement augmentation was a cost-effective modality when a cutoff of €30,000, 181
Computed tomography (CT)-based techniques, 218
Conical screws, 74
Cortical screw, 89
cortical screw fixation, 89
cortical screws, 88
cortical screw systems, 90–94
– components, 88
– efficacy and complications, 89
Corticocancellous allograft, 191
cranial-caudal, 11
Criteria for vertebral body replacement, 156

## D

degenerative disease, 11
degenerative spine conditions, 124
Demineralised bone matrix [DBM], 191
DePuy Synthes chronOS® Bone Void Filler: Block, 195
DePuy Synthes chronOS® Bone Void Filler: Granules 195
DePuy Synthes chronOS® Bone Void Filler: Wedge, 196
DePuy Synthes Concorde® Bullet Ti, 49
DePuy Synthes COUGAR® LS Lateral Cage System, 139, 140
DePuy Synthes DBX® Demineralized Bone Matrix: Inject, 205
DePuy Synthes DBX® Demineralized Bone Matrix: Mix, 206
DePuy Synthes DBX® Demineralized Bone Matrix: Putty, 206
DePuy Synthes DBX® Demineralized Bone Matrix: Strip, 207
DePuy Synthes INSIGHT® Lateral Access System, 126
DePuy Synthes OPAL™ Spacer System, 31
DePuy Synthes Spine VIPER® Cortical Fix Screw System, 91

DePuy Synthes Spine XRL® Vertebral Body Replacement Device, 166, 167
DePuy Synthes SPOTLIGHT® Access System, 13
DePuy Synthes SYNFLATE™ Vertebral Balloon, 184
DePuy Synthes T-PAL™ Interbody Spacer System, 32
DePuy Synthes Vertebral Body Balloon (VBB), 185
DePuy Synthes VERTECEM® Bone Cement, 186
DePuy Synthes VIPER® F2 Facet Fixation System, 99
DePuy Synthes VIPER® MIS Spine System, 77
DePuy Synthes ViviGen® Cellular Bone Matrix, 207
design of femoral cortical rings, 26
double lead, 74
dual thread screws, 74

## E

Ectopic bone formation, 193
Electromyographic (EMG) neuromonitoring, 121
expandable, 159
expandable carbon fiber VBR devices, 166–170
Expandable interbody cages, 27
expandable interbody cages, 66–71, 142–143
expandable metal VBR devices, 171–176
expandable retractor systems, 17–20
Expandable systems, 11
expandable titanium vertebral body replacement (VBR), 158
Expandable VBR implants, 157

## F

Facet screws, 96
facet screw systems, 98–102
– components, 96
– outcomes, 96–98
fiberoptic light system, 121
fibular strut, 156
fixed *versus* expandable systems, 11
flat blade, 21
flexion–extension movements of the lumbar spine, 105

Floppy retraction tower, 12
Floppy towers, 12
Fluoroscopic image of cannulated
pedicle screws, 8

## G

Globus Medical AFFIRM® Curved
Vertebral Compression Fracture
System, 187
Globus Medical ALTERA™
Interbody Cage, 67
Globus Medical CALIBER®
Interbody Cage, 68
Globus Medical CALIBER®-L, 142
Globus Medical CREO MCS™
Midline Cortical Stabilization
System, 92
Globus Medical CREO MIS™
Posterior Stabilization System,
78
Globus Medical FORGE® Oblique
Allograft Spacer, 63
Globus Medical FORTIFY® I
Corpectomy Spacer System, 171,
172
Globus Medical FORTIFY® I-R
Expandable Corpectomy Spacer
System, 168
Globus Medical FORTIFY® I-R
Static Corpectomy Spacer
System, 161
Globus Medical InterContinental®
LLIF Plate-Spacer System, 146,
147
Globus Medical LATIS® Interbody
Cage, 69
Globus Medical MARS™ 3V
Minimal Access Retractor
System, 126
Globus Medical MARS™ Minimal
Access Retractor System, 18
Globus Medical PLYMOUTH®
Thoracolumbar Plate System,
148
Globus Medical RISE®-L, 143
Globus Medical SHIELD® Vertebral
Compression Fracture System,
188
Globus Medical SUSTAIN® Arch, 50
Globus Medical SUSTAIN®-O, 34
Globus Medical SUSTAIN®-O TPS,
59
Globus Medical SUSTAIN®-R Arch,
33
Globus Medical SUSTAIN®-R Small
and Small Narrow, 35
Globus Medical SUSTAIN® Small
and Small Narrow, 51

Globus Medical TransContinental®,
133, 134
Globus Medical TransContinental®
titanium plasma spray (TPS),
141
Globus Medical ZYFUSE® Facet
Fixation System, 100

## H

horizontal cylinders (HCs), 26

## I

instrumentation, 96
interbody cage, 6
 – geometry
 – – expandable cages, 27
 – – standard cages, 26–27
 – materials, 27–28
 – overview, 26
interspinous fixation device
components, 104
interspinous fixation devices
(IFDs), 104
Interspinous fixation device with
clamps, 104

## J

Jamshidi trocar, 6

## K

K2M ALEUTIAN® AN and AN
Oblique Interbody Systems, 36
K2M ALEUTIAN® Lateral Interbody
System, 135
K2M ALEUTIAN® TLIF 2, 37
K2M CAPRI® Corpectomy Cage
System, 173
K2M CAPRI® Small 3D Static
Corpectomy Cage System, 164,
165
K2M CASCADIA™ AN, 52, 53
K2M CASCADIA™ Lateral, 138
K2M CASCADIA™ TL, 54
K2M CAYMAN® Minimally Invasive
Plate System, 149
K2M EVEREST® Minimally Invasive
Spinal System, 79
K2M RAVINE® Lateral Access
System, 128
K2M SANTORINI® Large
Corpectomy Cage System
Expandable Implant, 169, 170
K2M SANTORINI® Large
Corpectomy Cage System Solid
Implant, 162

K2M SERENGETI® Minimally
Invasive Retractor System, 22
K2M Terra Nova® Minimally
Invasive Access System, 23
K2M VENADO® Bone Graft System,
196
K2M VENADO® Foam Strips Bone
Graft System, 197
K2M VENADO® Granules Bone
Graft System, 197
K2M VESUVIUS® DBM Putty 100
Osteobiologic System, 208
K2M VESUVIUS® Demineralized
Fibers Osteobiologic System,
198
K2M VESUVIUS® Demineralized
Sponge Osteobiologic System,
198
K2M VEUVIUS® DBM Putty
Osteobiologic System, 208
K2M VIKOS® Shafts Allograft
System, 213
K2M VIKOS® Void Fillers Allograft
System, 214
Kyphoplasty, 180
kyphoplasty, 181
kyphoplasty procedure with
balloon dilation, 181

## L

Lateral decubitus positioning for
MIS lateral approach, 121
lateral fixation systems, 145–154
Lateral fluoroscopic image of the
interbody cage, 7
lateral interbody cages
 – expandable interbody cages,
142–143
 – static metal interbody cages,
138
 – static mixed composition
interbody cages, 139–141
 – static PEEK lateral interbody
cages, 133–137
lateral lumbar interbody fusion
(LLIF), 121
lateral lumbar interbody fusions
(LLIFs), 145
lateral retractor systems, 126–131
lumbar plexus branches, 121

## M

medial-lateral planes, 11
Medtronic Capstone PTC™, 60
Medtronic CD Horizon®
Longitude® II Multilevel

Percutaneous Fixation System, 80
Medtronic CD Horizon® Solera® Cortical Fixation Spinal System, 93
Medtronic CD Horizon® Solera® Spinal System, 81
Medtronic CD Horizon® Solera® Voyager Spinal System, 82
Medtronic Elevate™, 70, 71
Medtronic MAST® Quadrant™ Retractor System, 19
Medtronic METRx® II System, 14
Medtronic StealthStation™ S8 Surgical Navigation System, 220
Metal, 157
midline lumbar fusion (MIDLF), 88
Minimally invasive cortical screw placement, 88
Minimally invasive spine (MIS), 1
– closure and postoperative care, 8
– disk space preparation, 5–6
– interbody cage placement, 6
– lateral approach
–– complications, 123
–– surgical anatomy, 120
–– surgical technique, 120–123
– posterior approach
–– surgical anatomy, 4–9
– supplemental fixation, 6–8
– transforaminal lumbar interbody fusion, 4–5
minimally invasive transforaminal lumbar interbody fusion, 28
minimally invasive transforaminal lumbar interbody fusions (MIS TLIFs), 27
MIS. See Minimally invasive spine (MIS)
Monoplanar screws, 74

N

Navigation systems, 218
nonexpandable implants, 159
NuVasive Affix® II Spinous Process Plate Device, 108
NuVasive Attrax® Putty, 199
NuVasive CoRoent® Large Contoured, 38
NuVasive CoRoent® Large Narrow and Wide, 39
NuVasive CoRoent® Large Oblique (LO) Interbody Cage Device, 40, 136
NuVasive CoRoent® Large Tapered Interbody Cage Device, 41
NuVasive CoRoent® MAS® PLIF, 42

NuVasive Formagraft® Collagen Bone Graft Matrix, 199
NuVasive Integrated Global Alignment, 221
NuVasive MAS® PLIF Platform, 94
NuVasive MaXcess® 4 Access System, 129
NuVasive MaXcess® Mas® PLIF Access System, 24
NuVasive MaXcess® Mas® TLIF 2 Main Access System, 25
NuVasive Osteocel® Pro Allograft Cellular Bone Matrix, 200
NuVasive Propel™ Demineralized Bone Matrix Fibers, 209
NuVasive Propel™ Demineralized Bone Matrix Putty, 209
NuVasive Reline® Posterior Fixation System, 83
NuVasive SpheRx® DBR III Spinal System, 84
NuVasive SpheRx® II Anterior System, 150
NuVasive Traverse® Anterior Plate System, 151, 152
NuVasive Triad Allograft Spacer, 64
NuVasive X-CORE® 2 Expandable VBR, 175, 176
NuVasive X-CORE® Expandable VBR, 174

O

open boxes (OBs), 26
Open box interbody cage, 27
orthopaedic balloons, 181
OsteoMed PrimaLOK™ SP Interspinous Fusion System, 109
osteoporotic thoracolumbar compression fractures, 181
osteoporotic thoracolumbar fractures, 159
Osteoporotic VCFs, 180
Oswestry Disability Index (ODI), 9, 124, 182

P

Paradigm Spine Coflex® Interlaminar Technology, 110, 111
pedicle screw, 74
– based retractor systems, 22–25
– based systems, 11–12
– components, 73–75
– constructs, 75
pedicle-screw–based systems, 12
pedicle screw fixation, 89
pedicle screw placement, 74

pedicle screws, 88
percutaneous cement augmentation systems, 180–188
Percutaneous pedicle screws, 6
percutaneous pedicle screw systems, 76–86
– complications, 75
– pedicle screw components, 73–75
– pedicle screw constructs, 75
permanent neural injury, 120
Polyetheretherketone (PEEK), 27
polyetheretherketone (PEEK), 157
polymethyl methacrylate (PMMA), 181
Posterior interbody cages
– expandable interbody cages, 66–71
– interbody cage geometry–expandable cages, 27
– interbody cage geometry–standard cages, 26–27
– interbody cage materials, 27–28
– interbody cage overview, 26
– minimally invasive transforaminal lumbar interbody fusion, 28
– static allograft interbody cages, 63–65
– static carbon fiber interbody cages, 29–47
– static metal interbody cages, 48–56
– static mixed composition interbody cages, 57–62
posterior lumbar interbody cages, 26
posterior lumbar interbody fusion [PLIF], 192
posterior parasagittal technique, 4
Posterior Retractor Systems, 96
posterior retractor systems
– complications, 11–12
– expandable retractor systems, 17–20
– fixed versus expandable systems, 11
– flat blade, 21
– pedicle-screw–based retractor systems, 22–25
– pedicle-screw–based systems, 11–12
– retractor components, 11
– static retractor systems, 13–17
prevertebral swelling, 193

Q

qualityadjusted life year (QALY), 181

## R

radiopaque titanium, 158
randomized controlled trial (RCT), 181
recombinant human bone morphogenetic protein-2 (rhBMP-2), 122
recombinant human bone morphogenetic protein [rhBMP], 191
Reduction towers, 12
removal of the ligamentum flavum, 7
Retraction systems, 11
retractor components, 11
rget trajectory for pedicle screw placement, 73
RTI Surgical BacFuse® Spinous Process Fusion Plate System, 112
RTI surgical bullet-tip, 43
RTI Surgical Clarity® MIS Port System, 15
RTI Surgical Cross-Fuse® II PEEK VBR/IBF System, 137
RTI Surgical Lat-Fuse® Lateral Plate System, 153
RTI Surgical MaxFuse® PEEK VBR System, 163
RTI Surgical Streamline® MIS Spinal Fixation System, 85
RTI surgical T-Plus™, 44

## S

Screw–plate constructs, 145
Screw trajectories, 88
SeaSpine Allograft, 215
SeaSpine Compressible Bone Matrix, 200
SeaSpine Hollywood™, 45
SeaSpine Hollywood™ NanoMetalene®, 61
SeaSpine iPassage™ MIS Retractor, 20
SeaSpine OsteoSparx® and OsteoSparx® C, 210
SeaSpine OsteoSurge® 100, 211
SeaSpine OsteoSurge® 300 and 300 c, 211
SeaSpine Spine Pure Strip Allograft, 210
SeaSpine Spinous Process Fixation System, 113
SeaSpine Ventura™, 46
SeaSpine Ventura™ NanoMetalene, 62
Serial dilators, 121
single-incision approaches, 121

spine-specific patient-reported measures, 124
spinous process fixation systems, 106–116
– interspinous fixation device components, 104
Standard pedicle screw placement, 97
Standard retraction tower, 12
static allograft interbody cages, 63–65
static carbon fiber interbody cages, 29–47
static metal interbody cages, 48–56, 138
static metal VBR devices, 164–165
static mixed composition interbody cages, 57–62, 139–141
static PEEK lateral interbody cages, 133–137
static PEEK VBR devices, 160–163
static retractor systems, 13–17
Stryker LITe® Midline retractor, 21
Stryker Tritanium® PL, 55
Stryker UniVise® Spinous Process Fixation Plate System, 114
Surgical indications for facet screws, 96
Surgical indications for interspinous fixation devices, 104
Surgical indications for percutaneous pedicle screws, 73
Surgical indications for vertebral plates, 145
Surgical navigation systems, 218–222

## T

Titanium, 27
traditional cancellous pedicle screws, 88
Transfacet pedicle technique, 97
transfacet pedicle techniques, 96
transforaminal lumbar interbody fusion (TLIF), 124, 192
transforming growth factor-beta (TGF-?), 192
translaminar transfacet, 96
Translaminar transfacet technique, 97
Trial sizers, 6
tricalcium phosphate (TCP), 192
tricortical iliac bone crest, 156
Tubular dilators, 11

## U

unilateral or bilateral percutaneous balloon kyphoplasty, 182

## V

Vascular injury with LLIF, 123
vertebral arthrodesis, 26
vertebral body replacement (VBR), 156
vertebral body replacement devices
– classification
–– composition, 157–158
–– design, 157
– expandable carbon fiber VBR devices, 166–170
– expandable metal VBR devices, 171–176
– static metal VBR devices, 164–165
– static PEEK VBR devices, 160–163
vertebral body replacement (VBR) implant, 157
vertebral compression fracture, 180
Vertebral compression fractures (VCFs), 180
vertebral compression fractures (VCFs), 156
Vertebroplasty, 180
vertical rings (VRs), 26
Visual Analog Scale (VAS), 9, 124, 181

## Z

Ziehm Imaging Vision RFD 3D, 222
Zimmer Biomet AccuVision® Minimally Invasive Spinal Exposure System, 129
Zimmer Biomet ALPINE XC™ Adjustable Fusion System, 115
Zimmer Biomet ASPEN® MIS Fusion System, 116
Zimmer Biomet Cellentra® Advanced Allograft, 215
Zimmer Biomet CONCERO™ Facet Screw System, 101
Zimmer Biomet CopiOs® Bone Void Filler, 201
Zimmer Biomet Fortis PLIF Allograft Interbody Spacer, 65
Zimmer Biomet Indux™ Cancellous Sponge and Cortical Strip, 201

Zimmer Biomet InterGro® DBM, 212

Zimmer Biomet LDR FacetBRIDGE™ Facet Fixation System, 102

Zimmer Biomet PathFinder NXT™ Pedicle Screw Fixation System, 86

Zimmer Biomet PlatFORM™ CM Osteoconductive Collagen Mineral Bone Graft Matrix, 204

Zimmer Biomet PrimaGen Advanced™ Allograft, 216

Zimmer Biomet Pro Osteon® Bone Graft Substitute: Block, 202

Zimmer Biomet Pro Osteon® Bone Graft Substitute: Granules, 203

Zimmer Biomet Pro Osteon® Bone Graft Substitute: Wedge, 203

Zimmer Biomet Puros® Demineralized Bone Matrix (DBM), 212, 213

Zimmer Biomet Timberline® Lateral Fusion System, 131

Zimmer Biomet Timberline® MPF Lateral Modular Plate Fixation System, 154

Zimmer Biomet TM Ardis® Interbody System, 56

Zimmer Biomet Viewline™ Tube Retraction System, 16

Zimmer Biomet Zyston® Curve Interbody Spacer System, 47